100 Questions & Answers About Your Sports Injury

Thomas M. Howard, MD

Program Director
VCU—Fairfax Family Practice Sports Medicine Fellowship
Fairfax, VA

Gary WK Ho, MD

Assistant Program Director
VCU—Fairfax Family Practice Sports Medicine Fellowship
Fairfax, VA

Edward Josiah Lewis, MD

Sports Medicine Fellow
VCU—Fairfax Family Practice Sports Medicine Fellowship
Fairfax, VA

JONES AND BARTLETT PUBLISHERS
Sudbury, Massachusetts
BOSTON   TORONTO   LONDON   SINGAPORE

World Headquarters
Jones and Bartlett Publishers
40 Tall Pine Drive
Sudbury, MA 01776
978-443-5000
info@jbpub.com
www.jbpub.com

Jones and Bartlett Publishers
Canada
6339 Ormindale Way
Mississauga, Ontario L5V 1J2
Canada

Jones and Bartlett Publishers
International
Barb House, Barb Mews
London W6 7PA
United Kingdom

Jones and Bartlett's books and products are available through most bookstores and online booksellers. To contact Jones and Bartlett Publishers directly, call 800-832-0034, fax 978-443-8000, or visit our website, www.jbpub.com.

Substantial discounts on bulk quantities of Jones and Bartlett's publications are available to corporations, professional associations, and other qualified organizations. For details and specific discount information, contact the special sales department at Jones and Bartlett via the above contact information or send an email to specialsales@jbpub.com.

Cover Credits
Left photo (pitcher): © Bryan Eastham/
　ShutterStock, Inc.
Top right photo (runner): © LiquidLibrary

Middle right photo (football player): © Ron
　Chapple/Thinkstock/Alamy Images
Bottom right photo (tennis player): © Galina
　Barskaya/ShutterStock, Inc.

Production Credits
Executive Publisher: Christopher Davis
Associate Editor: Kathy Richardson
Production Director: Amy Rose
Production Editor: Daniel Stone
Marketing Associate: Rebecca Wasley

Manufacturing and Inventory Controller:
　Therese Connell
Composition: Appingo
Cover Design: Jonathan Ayotte
Printing and Binding: Malloy, Inc.
Cover Printing: Malloy, Inc.

The authors, editor, and publisher have made every effort to provide accurate information. However, they are not responsible for errors, omissions, or for any outcomes related to the use of the contents of this book and take no responsibility for the use of the products and procedures described. Treatments and side effects described in this book may not be applicable to all people; likewise, some people may require a dose or experience a side effect that is not described herein. Drugs and medical devices are discussed that may have limited availability controlled by the Food and Drug Administration (FDA) for use only in a research study or clinical trial. Research, clinical practice, and government regulations often change the accepted standard in this field. When consideration is being given to use of any drug in the clinical setting, the health care provider or reader is responsible for determining FDA status of the drug, reading the package insert, and reviewing prescribing information for the most up-to-date recommendations on dose, precautions, and contraindications, and determining the appropriate usage for the product. This is especially important in the case of drugs that are new or seldom used.

Library of Congress Cataloging-in-Publication Data
Howard, Thomas M.
　100 questions & answers about your sports injury / Thomas M. Howard, Garry
Wk Ho, Edward Josiah Lewis.
　　p. cm.
　Includes bibliographical references and index.
　ISBN-13: 978-0-7637-4638-4
　ISBN-10: 0-7637-4638-X
　1. Sports injuries--Miscellanea. 2. Sports medicine--Miscellanea. I. Ho,
Garry Wk. II. Lewis, Edward Josiah. III. Title. IV. Title: One hundred
questions and answers about your sports injury.
　RD97.H69 2008
　617.1'027--dc22
　　　　　　　　　　　　2007039685
6048

Printed in the United States of America
11 10 09 08　　　10 9 8 7 6 5 4 3 2

This book is dedicated to our families, who have endured endless nights and weekends alone while we were fieldside or courtside covering various sport activities in the practice of sports medicine.

Additionally, this book is dedicated to the countless patients we have encountered and helped over the years. Each patient interaction is an opportunity to help the patient return to his or her chosen activity, but also an educational opportunity for us.

Introduction   **vii**

Part 1: General Information   *1*

Questions 1-20 provides general information about sports-related injuries.
- Which sports injuries are more common in female athletes, and how can I prevent them?
- If I have diabetes, high blood pressure, or another chronic medical condition, can I safely participate in sports and exercise?
- How do I treat and prevent muscle spasms and cramps?
- Are there some general things I can do to prevent sports-related injuries?

Part 2: Head, Face, and Neck Injuries   *33*

Questions 21-31 discuss injuries to the head, face, and neck area and what to do about them.
- What is a concussion and what should I do about it?
- What should I do about headaches?
- What do I do about nosebleeds?
- What should I do about facial injuries?

Part 3: Upper Extremity Injuries   *51*

Questions 32-47 go into detail about injuries to the upper extremities and remedies to take care of them.
- What is shoulder impingement or rotator cuff tendonitis, and what should I do about it?
- What should I do if my shoulder pops out of socket?
- What is a frozen shoulder, and what should I do about it?

Part 4: Trunk Injuries   *75*

Questions 48-55 provide information on injuries to the trunk area.
- I got hit in the ribs, and they really hurt; what should I do now?
- I got hit in the abdomen, and it really hurts; what should I do now?

- What are side stitches, and what should I do about them?
- What should I do about my back pain?

Part 5: *Lower Extremity Injuries*   *87*

Questions 56-76 discuss injuries to the lower extremities and how to deal with them.
- What should I do about my groin pull?
- What is a sports hernia, and what should be done about it?
- What should I do about my hip pain?
- What should I do if my hip clicks, pops, or crackles?

Part 6: *Sport-Specific Injuries*   *127*

Questions 77-100 discuss sport specific injuries.
- What are the most common injuries in baseball, and how can I prevent them?
- What are the most common running injuries, and how can I prevent them?
- What are the most common basketball injuries, and how can I prevent them?
- What are the most common skiing and snowboarding injuries, and how can I prevent them?

Exercises	**169**
Glossary	**205**
Bibliography	**209**
Index	**211**

Much of our current news in America speaks of the growing trend of inactivity and obesity that affects up to one-third of our population, and this number is increasing. In the face of this concerning trend, there is another group of Americans that are active—and perhaps overactive—in various recreational and occupational activities. This includes the three-season youth athlete, the athlete participating and focusing on one sport year-round, the weekend adult athlete, and the occupational athlete. Unfortunately, many of these well-meaning individuals often find their sport to be less than enjoyable. Additionally, with growing medical costs, people are looking for self-help guides to help with the diagnosis and home management of the common problems encountered in their chosen sport or activity.

This book is not a substitute for appropriate medical evaluation and treatment, but is meant to assist those contemplating a new sport or encountering minor problems associated with their current sport activity.

This book represents the translation of many common patient education discussions we have had over the years. Our goal has always been to explain common medical conditions in terms easily understood as to the cause, the recovery, the rehabilitation process, and prevention strategies.

There are numerous, and perhaps too many, internet-based sources to learn about these various conditions. These sources include various clinical practice guidelines and other well-known professional organizations. Some of these references are discussed in the last question of this book.

It is our wish that you find this book helpful and that it makes you a more educated medical consumer. Fitness is a lifelong pursuit, both physically and emotionally, and we hope this will help those active individuals continue to stay active. Darwin had it right: "Only the fittest survive".

PART ONE

General Information

Which sports injuries are more common in female
athletes, and how can I prevent them?

I find it difficult to breathe when
I exercise. What's wrong with me?

How do I treat and prevent
muscle spasms and cramps?

More . . .

1. Which sports injuries are more common in female athletes, and how can I prevent them?

Although the overall risk of the various injuries in sports is more related to the sport, equipment, and terrain or surface, there are some problems that are more common in the female competitor. Among these are injuries to the anterior cruciate ligament (ACL) of the knee and the incidence of patello-femoral pain syndrome. Patellofemoral pain syndrome is more completely discussed in Question 62. Additionally, a condition unique to female athletes is the female athlete triad.

The ACL resists forward movement of the tibia (lower leg) on the femur (thigh). Female athletes have at least a three times greater risk of ACL injury than their male counterparts in sports such as soccer and basketball. About 70–80% of ACL injuries occur during noncontact activities, e.g., landing from a jump or cutting and stopping. Typical sports in which ACL injuries occur include soccer, basketball, and volleyball.

There are multiple theories about why there is an increased incidence of noncontact ACL injuries in young women. Anatomic predisposing factors may include a wider pelvis, a more **valgus** (angled outward) knee (knocked-knee), a narrower femoral notch (the space where the ACL is located) and/or a smaller ligament diameter. Additionally, it has been suggested that there may be a hormonal influence with more ACL ruptures occurring during certain points of the menstrual cycle.

In an activity that stresses the ACL, the hamstrings work as a dynamic resistance to forward translation of the tibia. In women, the activation of the hamstrings appears to be delayed relative to male athletes, placing the ACL in jeopardy during these activities. Additionally, women tend to land with their knees in more **extension** (more straight) and more flat footed. When involved in cutting activities, they are more erect than their male counterparts. With all of the above, women tend

Valgus

Movement or posturing of a limb in which the part farther from the center of the body is farther from the midline.

Extension

Movement of a joint moving away from the body or straightening.

to be more ligament-dependent for stability than men, and their functional differences with landing and cutting/pivoting put more stress on the ACL.

Prevention strategies focus on rehabilitation to improve hamstring strength and tone as well as landing and cutting drills. Women who are involved in higher-risk sports should train year-round. Landing and cutting drills should focus on two-foot landing with the knee bent and going into a crouch, rounded turns rather that planting and pivoting, and a three-step stop. Additionally, single-leg balance drills add further stability during high-risk activities.

The female athlete triad identifies a collection of three diagnoses—osteoporosis, amenorrhea (absence of menstrual periods) and stress fractures. In fact, these three diagnoses are very interrelated and not separate diagnoses. The underlying theme for this collection of problems is inadequate energy intake (nutrition) for the level of activity. A female athlete training hard and trying to restrict calories or just not increasing caloric intake enough will stress her body and the body's initial response will be the irregularity and then the cessation of menstrual periods. Part of this menstrual irregularity and loss is related to a low estrogen state. This, combined with poor nutritional intake, slows the development of new bone that should be occurring up to the age of 30. In fact, calcium may be leached out of the bone. As this progresses, along with the bone stress from her chosen exercise or sport, stress fractures will follow. The prevention strategy is simple—consume adequate calories for the level of exercise. This is usually around 1200–1500 calories.

2. If I have diabetes, high blood pressure, or another chronic medical condition, can I safely participate in sports and exercise?

Exercise plays a key role in health maintenance and disease prevention as well; it is a critical component in the management of most medical problems. There are very few medical conditions where exercise in some form is not recommended.

Before considering an exercise program in the presence of medical problems, you should seek the advice of your doctor. In some, a preexercise examination to include up-to-date lab assessment, electrocardiogram, and even stress testing are considered. You should consider evaluation for a preexercise stress test if you have significant cardiovascular risk factors. These risk factors include being older than 40 in men and older than 50 in women, presence of diabetes, high blood pressure, elevated cholesterol, a family history of early heart disease (especially in close relatives like brothers, sisters, or parents), and a desire to take on a vigorous exercise routine.

Walking is a great form of exercise. Brisk walking on a soft surface for 30 minutes most days of the week is ideal. Those with bad arthritis of the hips or knees should consider other lower impact aerobic activity like swimming, cycling, or using an elliptical trainer or stair machine. Diabetics with nerve damage in their feet need to be especially cautious about their foot care, especially if they choose to run or expose themselves to temperature extremes. Those who have busy lifestyles can increase their activity with everyday chores and activities. Parking in the back of the parking lot and taking the stairs if we have to ascend two floors or fewer or descend four or fewer are everyday things we can do to increase our activity.

In additional to aerobic training, people should also add resistance training; light weight lifting, using the major muscles of the upper and lower extremities and doing core strengthening exercises 2 days per week; and a regular program of stretching most days of the week. Exercise or physical activity should not be looked upon as a burden, but as a necessary part of your daily schedule.

3. I'm pregnant and still want to exercise or play sports; can I do so safely?

There are many potential health benefits to exercising while pregnant, including maintaining your fitness level, improved appreciation of your body and self-esteem, and the avoidance of excessive weight gain from pregnancy.

However, there have been many concerns with exercising and sports participation while pregnant. Some of these concerns have been supported and others have been shown to be invalid by both medical experts and research studies. These include concerns regarding potential overheating and hormone imbalances, as well as the shunting of blood and nutrients away from the developing baby. In the past, doctors have been concerned about possible birth defects, interfering with the baby's growth, low birth weight, preterm labor, miscarriages, and other complications as a result of exercising while pregnant. But there is certainly good news if you want to exercise: more than 70 studies and expert recommendations since 1985 have shown that exercising and playing sports while pregnant can be safe and even good for both the baby and the mother-to-be.

The amazing thing is that the human body adapts to both pregnancy and exercise demands. More recent studies have shown that preterm labor, premature rupture of membranes, gestational diabetes, varicose veins, and back pain are actually decreased in pregnant women who exercise moderately. High-intensity exercise may lead to a moderate decrease in birth weight, but moderate levels of exercise actually enhance birth weight and improve the baby's alertness and mood after delivery.

> *The amazing thing is that the human body adapts to both pregnancy and exercise demands.*

If you wish to exercise, you should always check with your physician first. Some important tips and considerations include the following:

1. Exercise at mild to moderate levels of intensity, three times a week.

2. Exercise at intensity levels similar to your pre–pregnancy levels, or at a moderate level of intensity. You can tell that you are exercising at moderate intensity by doing the "talk test": make sure you can still talk aloud in complete sentences while you are exercising.

3. Avoid dehydration by making sure you hydrate before, during, and after exercise with sports drinks as well as water. Start with drinking 1 pint of liquid before and 1 cup of liquid every 20 minutes during exercise, even if you are not thirsty. You can then adjust depending on how you personally process fluids.

4. Make sure you take in enough calories to maintain the energy that you and your baby need. Pregnancy itself requires an additional 300 calories a day (and lactation requires 500 additional calories a day), but you'll need more than this, since you will be using up calories exercising. On average, most women should gain 25–35 pounds over the entire pregnancy, although this may vary. Check with your physician and together you can set weight-gain goals.

5. Wear appropriate clothing and avoid exercising in hot, humid environments.

6. Make sure you get plenty of rest and time to recuperate from exercise, especially later in your pregnancy.

7. If any activity causes pain, stop and consult your physician.

8. Avoid activities where you might lose your balance, fall, or get hit by something or someone, like ice hockey, skiing, kickboxing, soccer, or horseback riding.

9. Avoid ballistic movements, activities in which you lie flat on your back, and, after 16 weeks of gestational age, activities in which you hold your breath and strain. When lifting weights, avoid straining your back, and always use good breathing technique.

10. Pregnant women should absolutely *never* participate in scuba diving, skydiving, or any exercise at high altitudes.

There are times and situations in which a pregnant woman should absolutely not exercise or participate in sports. These include those with pregnancy-related high blood pressure, incompetent cervix, vaginal bleeding, placental problems, and those with current, active problems with preterm labor, premature rupture of membranes, or interference in the baby's growth. Consult your physician if there is any doubt or question whether you should exercise whatsoever.

Situations in which a pregnant woman may exercise under the close supervision of a physician include chronic high blood pressure, **anemia**, heart disease, lung disorders, diabetes, and thyroid problems. Again, consult your physician.

4. I've got a cold or the flu and still want to exercise or play sports. What should I do?

In all but the mildest of cases of upper respiratory infections (**URI**), like the cold or the flu, the athlete should consult a physician before continuing to exercise or play sports. A URI can worsen and last longer than needed if the athlete does not rest and hydrate adequately. Also, if the athlete is participating in sports with others, there is a risk of spreading the disease to teammates and other athletes.

In general, athletes with a fever should not exercise or participate in competitive sports. A fever is defined as a core body temperature of 100.4°F (38°C). The most accurate temperature measurement is a rectal temperature. Oral temperature is acceptable and more accurate than axillary or forehead skin temperatures. Heat injury, like heat exhaustion and heatstroke (which is life threatening), are more likely in athletes with a fever. Fever can significantly increase the workload on the cardiovascular (heart and blood vessels) and pulmonary (lungs, airways, and breathing) systems. Fever makes it easier for muscles to fatigue and for the body to become dehydrated.

Anemia
Low blood count; often from iron deficiency or blood loss.

URI
Upper respiratory infection; a cold.

Those with gastrointestinal (stomach or bowel) illnesses, especially those with nausea, vomiting, or diarrhea, should not participate either. The fluid and electrolyte imbalances can be very uncomfortable or even dangerous to the athlete.

In addition, some athletes getting over a viral infection may have a myocarditis (a rare type of heart muscle inflammation). Although rare, strenuous exercise may be dangerous in these individuals, leading to life-threatening heart rhythms.

Many experts agree that sports performance declines in athletes with URIs. Agility and balance are affected by URIs, and the athlete should consider reducing the intensity of exercise or not participating in competitive sports while recovering from a URI.

Athletes need to be aware of the possibility they may come down with mono (infectious mononucleosis), which is a viral condition that affects the muscles, lymph nodes, liver, and spleen. In general, if one has mono, he or she should not participate. There are many concerns, but the most frightening one is the risk of rupturing the spleen and causing life-threatening internal bleeding. Although the amount of recovery time is controversial, most experts agree that an athlete with mono should be restricted from participation for at least 21 days. Those playing in contact sports should be restricted from contact for 28 days. All athletes with mono should be under the care of a physician, who will check to see if the spleen is enlarged, and if it is, the physician will also check to make sure that it returns to normal before allowing the athlete to return to sport. The method with which the physician assesses the spleen is controversial and may include a physical exam or an ultrasound.

Many experts recommend using the "neck check" test in deciding whether an athlete with a URI should participate. If symptoms are located above the neck, then the athlete may cautiously exercise or participate at half the usual intensity or speed. Above-the-neck symptoms include stuffy or runny nose, sneezing, or scratchy throat with *no* fever, chills, or sweats. If these symptoms clear and the athlete feels better, then the exercise intensity can be gradually increased. If the athlete feels worse, he or she should rest. Athletes with below–the–neck symptoms should not participate. These symptoms include fever (temp greater than 100.4° f), aching muscles, a hacking cough with phlegm, nausea, vomiting, or diarrhea.

In general, athletes with a very mild URI, no below-the-neck symptoms, and no fever may participate under the supervision of a physician or other health care professional. Some key considerations include:

1. Athletes feeling as if they may be getting sick should reduce the intensity and duration of their exercise for 1 or 2 days.
2. Exercise at mild to moderate levels of intensity only; avoid more strenuous activity.
3. Being sick means you need more fluids. Avoid dehydration by making sure you hydrate before, during, and after exercise with sports drinks as well as water. Start with drinking 1 pint of liquid before and 1 cup of liquid every 20 minutes during exercise, even if you are not thirsty. You can then adjust depending on how you personally process fluids.
4. Being sick means you need more calories. Make sure you take in enough calories to maintain the energy that you need to both fight the URI and fuel your exercise.
5. Wear appropriate clothing and avoid exercising in hot, humid environments.
6. Being sick means you need more rest. Your body is busy enough fighting illness or infection. Make sure you get plenty of rest and time to recuperate from exercise.
7. If any activity causes pain, stop and consult your physician.

General Information

8. Avoid activities in which you might lose your balance, fall, or get hit by something or someone, like ice hockey, skiing, kickboxing, soccer, or horseback riding.

9. Avoid scuba diving, skydiving, or exercise at high altitudes.

10. Use over-the-counter acetaminophen (like Tylenol) for fever, muscle, and joint aches. Avoid using aspirin or medications containing antihistamines (found in many allergy medications). While this is controversial, consider being judicious about using nonsteroidal anti-inflammatory drugs (**NSAIDs**) like ibuprofen and naproxen. Some over-the-counter cold remedies are banned by certain sports organizations; check with your coach, athletic trainer, physician, or sports official if you have any questions.

NSAID

Nonsteroidal anti-inflammatory drugs; e.g., naproxen, ibuprofen, etc.

5. How do I treat and prevent muscle spasms and cramps?

Muscle spasms and cramps are common problems associated with prolonged episodes of exercise. This could include running a marathon or triathlon or even a football or soccer game.

There is much controversy as to what really causes these exercise-associated cramps and spasm. Electrolyte problems and dehydration are often cited; however, in some scientific studies looking at this cause it was not found to be true. Certainly inadequate electrolyte and fluid intake and poor preexercise nutrition will contribute to the development of cramps. Additionally, it may be more common in warm temperatures likely associated with increased sweating.

More likely, cramps and spasms represent fatigued muscles that have been pushed to the extreme.

More likely, cramps and spasms represent fatigued muscles that have been pushed to the extreme. It is not uncommon that the players likely to suffer cramps are those running more or faster, such as linebackers, defensive backs, and running backs in football, or a midfielder or forward in soccer.

The first treatment for muscle spasms and cramps is prevention. Adequate conditioning for the proposed activity is the number one preventive, followed by adequate hydration and nutrition before and during athletic events. There are anecdotal reports for the success of pickle juice or electrolyte solutions for hydration and restoration of electrolytes and fluids. In the event of an acute spasm or cramp, the individual can stretch the affected muscle, which is often a calf, hamstring, or quadriceps (front of thigh). As soon as the cramp is improved, the individual should walk around to improve blood flow to the muscle and allow recovery. Occasionally, cramps not responding to aggressive treatment on the field or sidelines will need evaluation and treatment in the emergency room.

6. I find it difficult to breathe when I exercise. What's wrong with me?

Shortness of breath during exercise is a problem that affects many athletes and has many potential causes, including respiratory or heart-related (cardiac) causes, anemia (low blood count), and deconditioning. Shortness of breath associated with chest pain, fainting, or near fainting is concerning for a cardiac cause, and individuals with these symptoms should be evaluated by a physician prior to further exertion.

Two common respiratory causes of shortness of breath in athletes are exercise-induced bronchospasm and vocal cord dysfunction. The symptoms of exercise-induced bronchospasm (**EIB**), also known as exercise-induced asthma (EIA), are caused by an increase in airway resistance (resistance of airflow), which typically occurs with strenuous exercise and commonly includes cough, wheezing, and chest tightness, typically beginning 5–10 minutes after exercise. Up to 90% of asthmatics suffer from EIB, but many nonasthmatics and up to 15% of the general population experience these symptoms. It has been theorized that rapid water loss changes in the local environment in the bronchi (within the lung) causes constriction of the bronchioles, and that rapid temperature

EIB

Exercise-induced bronchospasm or wheezing.

changes may play a similar role. As such, EIB may be exacerbated during exercise in dry or cool environments and may be improved by exercising in a warm, humidified environment, covering the mouth and nose with a mask or scarf during cold weather exercise, avoiding allergens and pollutants, and warming up for at least 10 minutes before beginning vigorous exercise. EIB typically resolves spontaneously; however, your doctor may recommend a trial of inhaled albuterol 15–30 minutes prior to exercise, and other treatments are available. Other options for pretreatment include inhaled cromolyn (an anti-inflammatory agent) 30 minutes prior to exercise or a long-acting agent similar to albuterol called salmeterol. Those who have allergies and mild asthma with exercise aggravation may benefit with chronic management with anti-inflammatory medications like inhaled steroids (budesonide, triamcinolone acetonide, and fluticasone, to name a few) or a combination of salmeterol and a steroid called Salmeteral/Fluticasone. Athletes should be aware that salmeterol may cause aggravated exercise cramping.

Vocal cord dysfunction (VCD) is caused by abnormal closure of the vocal cords, particularly during inspiration, and may cause very similar symptoms to EIB or asthma. Vocal cord dysfunction does not respond to asthma medications and is frequently treated without success for some time before the appropriate diagnosis is made. Diagnosis is made by direct visualization of the vocal cords with a long, thin camera that is passed through the nose. VCD may be associated with irritants such as gastroesophageal reflux or chronic sinusitis/postnasal drip or allergies, and all of these factors should be treated if VCD is suspected. Your doctor may discuss other therapies and treatments with you if the diagnosis of VCD is made.

7. I get chest pain when I exercise. Should I be concerned?

Chest pain with exercise is a very concerning symptom because of the concern for cardiac causes of this pain. Exercise associated chest pains can be from cardiac, respiratory, gastro-intestinal, or even musculoskeletal causes. Although we will review common conditions and descriptions, if you experience exercise-related chest pain, you should be evaluated by your physician or in the emergency room.

Cardiac or heart-related chest pain is typically a pressure-like sensation in the central or left side of the chest. It may be associated with sweating, nausea, and light-headedness, and the pain may radiate to the left arm or jaw. Risk factors associated with cardiac problems include being a current smoker, a family history of heart disease in close blood relatives (brothers, sisters, and parents), diabetes, high blood pressure, obesity, in-activity, high cholesterol, and a history of prior heart problems. Again, individuals with a concern for heart-related chest pain should consider evaluation in the emergency room. Appropriate evaluation may include a good history and examination, blood work, electrocardiogram, and stress testing. The urgency of these tests really depends on the severity and frequency of the pain as well personal risk factors for heart disease. When in doubt, seek urgent evaluation.

Respiratory causes of exercise-associated chest pains may be associated with emphysema or asthma, or in rare cases throwing a clot to the lungs. Those with asthma may have more chest tightness, may have audible wheezing or cough spasm and a prior history of asthma or respiratory issues. For further discussion see Question 6. Acute clots in the lung cause acute symptoms of sharp chest pain and difficulty breathing. If you have acute clots, you may have a history of recent travel, surgery, or injury to the leg with immobilization. You may note leg swelling and pain and may have a family history of clots.

Stomach or gastrointestinal causes of chest pain with exercise are common. Heartburn or esophageal reflux is often aggravated by exercise. These individuals may have a prior experience with heartburn and even be on medications. The pain of heartburn is often a constant pressure-like pain in the central part of the chest with or without burning or a sour taste in the throat.

Chest pain may come from muscular or skeletal sources. Someone with chest pain may have a prior experience or a recent injury to the chest wall from a fall or being tackled or struck with a stick or object or the ground. This type of pain tends to be more sharp and localized to the area of injury. Often the pain gets worse with deep inspiration or coughing or when raising the arms overhead or with rotation of the trunk. These pains can be treated with relative rest from activities that aggravate the symptoms, application of ice for 15 minutes, or using ibuprofen or naproxen.

8. Are there some general things I can do to prevent sports-related injuries?

When addressing the issue of injury prevention, it is best to break injuries down into chronic or overuse and acute or traumatic injuries.

Extrinsic
Outside the body.

Intrinsic
Within the body.

Pronation
The motion of the forearm in which the palm rotates down or the foot becomes more flat.

To discuss the prevention of overuse injuries, we must review why we develop overuse injuries. Causes can be broken down into **extrinsic** (outside the body) and **intrinsic** (inside the body). We have more control over extrinsic issues than intrinsic issues, although awareness of intrinsic issues will allow one to train differently or choose different sports or activities. Intrinsic issues include muscle inflexibilities, weakness, short legs causing leg length issues, and excessive **pronation** (rolling of the feet). Extrinsic issues include the equipment we use, our technique for a given sport, training regimens, and where and when we train. It is not uncommon for people involved in certain activities do develop weakness in key muscle groups from repetitive use.

Equipment choices that cause injuries include worn-out shoes or the wrong shoes for runners, a tennis racket with strings that are too tight, or a grip that is too large for one's hand. Likewise, hard surfaces, such as concrete, can cause injuries for runners.

Acute and overuse injuries also can be related to poor technique in the performance of various motions we do in recreational and occupational repetitive activities. As we fatigue or as we try to push in competition, if we cheat on technique, we end up hurting ourselves.

So how do we prevent injury? Have properly fitted and appropriate equipment for a proposed activity. Know and practice appropriate technique even if it requires lessons or an independent observer. Train at an appropriate intensity and advance as tolerated and avoid the too much, too fast training program. Train with strength, endurance, and fitness exercises to prepare for any proposed occupational or recreational activity. Finally, listen to your body. If you are fatigued and you do not feel prepared to push yourself or recovered from your last exercise session, or you are feeling severe pain, back off and consider addressing some of the previous training issues or seek professional help.

9. When is it safe to resume exercise or playing sports after an injury or illness?

There are general guidelines for return to exercise or sports competition after injury or illness. These guidelines are just that and are really to protect the individual, as well as teammates and competitors.

Acute illness is often accompanied by fever, body aches, and fatigue, and it may have some focal symptoms depending on the illness as in cough, sore throat, vomiting, diarrhea, etc. (see Question 4). When someone is ill, a general guideline for whether to exercise and when to return is the "neck check." If the individual has symptoms below the neck manifested by fever > 100.4°F, muscle aching, severe cough, vomiting, or diarrhea, exercise should be suspended until these symptoms resolve. Upon return, it will generally take 2–3 days for every day off to get back to the previous level of fitness. If someone has symptoms above the neck as in no fever, congestion, and mild cough, then he or she may consider attempting to exercise. The individual should start out at 50% exertion, and if after 5 minutes he or she does not feel overly winded or fatigued, then he or she may exercise as tolerated.

Acute management of returning to exercise after injury will be discussed in Question 10. The general guideline for return to sports is that it is OK when the joint or body area has normal motion of the joint without pain and normal muscular strength. Individual recommendations will be covered in subsequent discussions.

A commonly used approach to controlling the damaging effects of early inflammation can be summarized with the acronym PRICEMM.

PRICEMM

A mnemonic for early management of injuries that stand for protection, relative rest, ice, compression, elevation, medications, and modalities.

10. In general, how should I initially treat my acute injury (immediate treatment tips)?

For almost all injuries, proper first aid and care in the first 1–3 days after sustaining an acute injury can make a big difference in how long it takes for you to recover from your injury. Damaged tissues will bleed and bruise, swell, and become irritated and inflamed, causing the area to be painful, red, and warm. This early inflammatory stage can be damaging before it progresses to the more healing, later stages of inflammation. However, inflammation is a normal part of the healing process. A commonly used approach to controlling the damaging effects of early inflammation can be summarized with the acronym **PRICEMM**. PRICEMM is designed to help speed healing by relieving pain, decreasing swelling and stiffness, and protecting the injured body part from further injury. PRICEMM stands for:

P— Protection: Injured tissue is susceptible to further damage, even from minor stresses. Pad, brace, tape, or splint the injured body part to support and protect it from further injury. A healthcare professional can help you with this, and may even recommend more aggressive protection including a cast. When in doubt, consult with a sports medicine or healthcare provider.

R— Relative rest: Rest helps protect the injured body part from further injury and save energy for the healing process. Limit use of the injured body part, avoiding any abusing activity. Complete immobilization, however, should be avoided unless recommended by a physician.

I— Ice: Cooling the injured body part decreases pain and inflammation in the surrounding area. You can use commercial ice or cold packs, but regular ice (crushed is best) or a package of frozen peas work just as well. Place a towel or other cloth between the skin and the ice pack to prevent frostbite. Apply the ice pack for 15 minutes. Do this at least three to four times a day for the first 1–3 days after an acute injury. Beware of overicing an area, which may cause skin burns or injure superficial nerves.

C— Compression: Gentle compression helps prevent and decrease swelling and pain. Make sure to use material that is elastic, as more rigid types of materials can cause further damage. Elastic bandages work well. The compression should be firm, but not painful, throbbing, or feel too tight. If the compression is too tight, remove the wrap and rewrap the injured body part slightly looser.

E— Elevation: Try to keep the injured body part elevated above the level of the heart to help control swelling. The higher the better.

M—Medications: Use over-the-counter acetaminophen as directed for pain relief. The use of nonsteroidal anti-inflammatory drugs (NSAIDs), such as ibuprofen or naproxen, is controversial (see Question 11). If NSAIDs are used for acute injuries, consider starting them 48–72 hours after the injury.

M—Modalities: Some physical therapy modalities, such as electrical stimulation and therapeutic ultrasound, are helpful in the short term. Make sure that any modalities you receive are provided or supervised by a qualified healthcare professional.

Approaches like PRICEMM work well for most injuries. You should see results within 48–72 hours. Gentle stretching, massage, warm compresses, and rehabilitation exercises may then be implemented. More severe injuries or cases not responding to PRICEMM should be evaluated by a healthcare professional. Consult your physician if you have any questions about your injury.

11. What OTC (over-the-counter) medication should I use for my injury—acetaminophen, ibuprofen, or something else?

There are many over-the-counter medications available for the treatment of sports injuries. They are best used as part of a more comprehensive treatment approach including rehabilitation exercises and PRICEMM (see Question 10).

There are several topical treatments that act to alleviate pain and introduce a cooling or warming effect to the site of injury. These may include ingredients like camphor, menthol, salicylates, capsaicin, and various oils and extracts. Topical treatments tend to be moderately effective in alleviating pain, and they may be useful in treating mild joint sprains and muscle strains. Side effects include skin irritation or a rash. This may be due to either a chemical irritation or an actual allergic reaction. Consult your healthcare professional if you have any type of reaction to these medications.

Over-the-counter oral medications can be very useful in alleviating pain from several different types of injuries. Many are also used to control fevers associated with other illnesses. These medications are generally processed by the liver and the kidneys. So, if you have liver or kidney problems, you should consult your healthcare professional before trying these medications. Acetaminophen, when used as directed, provides pain relief, but generally does not have a direct effect on inflammation and swelling. Acetaminophen is processed primarily by the liver. Nonsteroidal anti-inflammatory drugs (NSAIDs), such as ibuprofen or naproxen, provide pain relief as well, and they may have an effect on inflammation and swelling. However, if NSAIDs are used for acute injuries, consider starting them 48–72 hours after the injury, because early use may interfere with the healing process. NSAIDs are processed primarily by the kidneys, and overuse can stress kidneys and cause problems. Also, overuse can also lead to stomach problems including ulcers, but more commonly they cause mild discomfort. If you get abdominal discomfort from taking NSAIDs, consider taking them with food, or try a medication that treats stomach acid reflux (also available over the counter). If these don't help, consult your healthcare professional. If you are using NSAIDs for a more chronic condition such as arthritis (see Question 68), you might need to try several different NSAIDs, both over-the-counter as well as prescription varieties, to find the medication that works best for you. Every patient is unique, so work closely with your healthcare provider to find what works for you.

There are several other types of medications and preparations available outside of the United States. It is best to consult your healthcare provider before trying any of these alternatives. Also, the effectiveness of a particular medicine may or may not depend on how much of it you take. Once again, ask your pharmacist or healthcare provider if you think you might benefit from an increased dose. He or she may recommend increasing how much medication you take, changing the medication, or even a prescription-strength medication.

12. Are corticosteroid injections helpful for injuries? What are the risks of these injections?

Corticosteroid injections are commonly recommended and used to treat a multitude of conditions. These medications are thought to work by inhibiting the part of the immune system that causes inflammation and pain, although the way they do this is uncertain. In fact, whether or not the therapeutic effect of steroid injections is anti-inflammatory in nature has become controversial in the medical literature. Either way, many experts agree that steroid injections do have a role as an effective treatment modality for many problems. These include carpal tunnel syndrome, arthritis, tennis elbow, golfer's elbow, various types of tendonitis or tendinopathy, various types of **bursitis**, plantar fasciitis, frozen shoulder, Morton's neuroma, and ganglion cysts.

Bursitis

Inflammation of a bursa; from trauma or repetitive-friction causes.

However, steroid injections <u>should not be used alone</u> in the treatment of most conditions. By themselves, steroid injections tend to only relieve symptoms temporarily. Instead, they should be used in combination with other modes of therapy to address the underlying problem. This may include rehabilitation exercises, physical therapy modalities, splinting, or bracing.

Steroid injections use glucocorticoids (or corticosteroids), which are not the same as the anabolic steroids used to build muscle mass. Examples of some commonly used glucocorticoids include cortisone, dexamethasone, triamcinolone, and prednisone.

Steroid injections are not without potential risks. While relatively infrequent and kept to a minimum by the technique of a skilled clinician, complications may include thinning and discoloration of the skin, local infection, steroid flare, and damage to tendons and other tissues due to getting too many injections in the same area. Skin pigment changes and fat atrophy, when it occurs, usually will resolve in 6–9 months. Steroid flare is an acute exacerbation of the pain lasting 24–36 hours. The treatment of this is icing and pain management. Side effects of steroids include high blood pressure, diabetes, cataracts, agitation, and weight gain. These are far less common with local injections compared to steroids taken orally. People with certain medical conditions should not receive steroids; consult your healthcare provider if you have any questions about your medical conditions. Also, many people who receive steroids complain of some soreness.

If you think you may benefit from a steroid injection, consult a healthcare professional experienced in these injections. After receiving the injection, you may experience some soreness where the needle was inserted; cold packs may be helpful for this. The therapeutic effect of the steroid may not be evident until 3 days after the injection, and it may last anywhere from weeks to months. For the most part, you should limit the number of steroid injections you receive in a given area to no more than 3–4 treatments a year. More frequent injections have been associated with damage to surrounding tendons and other tissues.

13. How should I treat my scrape, cut, or puncture wound?

Minor and major injuries to the skin are common in everyday life as well with many recreational and sport activities. The first and foremost recommendation is to wash the injured area with warm water and soap with a mild abrasive cloth or such to remove any remaining debris and dirt. Puncture wounds should be thoroughly washed or soaked in warm water for 25 minutes.

After a good cleansing, a mild antibiotic ointment and a dressing should be applied. The type of dressing depends on the size of the wound and the location as well the risk of

General Information

further injury. Pain can be managed with ice and NSAIDs as discussed in Question 10.

Many of these wounds may increase the risk of tetanus infection and you should consider a booster immunization. Tetanus is associated with wounds contaminated with dirt or soil. Tetanus boosters are generally believed to be good for 10 years; however, in the presence of a dirty wound, 5 years is recommended. This booster shot should be administered within a week of such an injury.

Finally, you should observe the wound over the following week as it heals for signs of infections. This is usually manifested by increased pain, swelling, redness and warmth, and sometimes drainage. Wounds should not be treated with antibiotics preventively except for animal and human bites.

14. How should I treat my blisters?

Friction blisters are common in all age groups involved in all activities, but are more common in recreational activities. Because of rubbing between something pressed on the surface of the skin, a painful, fluid-filed bubble develops beneath the skin. Before the blister develops you may note some local irritation that is painful and red called a hot spot. If you aggressively treat the hot spot, you can avoid a painful blister.

Blisters are a result of friction from ill-fitting equipment and moisture, making the skin more susceptible to friction. The most common locations are the feet for most athletes, and then the hands. They often occur over bony prominences or under existing calluses. Repetitive motions also contribute to the development of these nagging injuries, which can become serious injuries if they become infected.

Prevention strategies begin with proper fit of athletic shoes and break-in periods for new shoes prior to extensive use in practice or games. The next strategy includes management of calluses and moisture control. Calluses should be pared down with an emery board, pumice stone, or paring blade. Moisture should be controlled with antiperspirant spray, polypropylene socks that are changed for each practice and game, or even a polypropylene sock liner under a game sock. Athletes with a tendency toward friction blisters over a particular bony prominence can pretreat the area with a lubricant like petroleum jelly or a moisturizer like.

Athletes should monitor themselves for the early development of hot spots, which is early inflammation of the skin prior to blister formation. Addressing these hot spots with padding, a moleskin doughnut, or adjustment of equipment may also alleviate the development of painful blisters. Ultra marathoners have been known to treat hot spots with tincture of benzoin and duct tape while in a race.

15. My performance is declining. I'm training harder and gaining less. What is wrong?

This question pertains to the diagnosis of overtraining.

Understanding the concept of overtraining requires a bit of a review of why we train and the body's response to this training. Overtraining is essentially the chronic fatigue of exercise.

Overtraining is essentially the chronic fatigue of exercise.

When you train or work out you are stressing your body to make it adapt so you can better respond to a similar physical stress in the future. A single episode or a training cycle requires a recovery period for this adaptation to occur. During this recovery time, you need adequate nutrition, hydration, sleep, and even emotional rest.

Fatigue is the body's response to hard training or other stress, indicating that you need to recover. So when you think of overtraining, think of all the causes of fatigue. Exercise has been said to be the great screening tool for disease. In general, if someone can exercise and feels good during and after then it is unlikely that the individual is overtrained or has any significant medical problem that may cause fatigue, like infections, cancer, anemia, electrolyte problems, thyroid problems, depression, or other conditions.

When we have just been training too hard, we become excessively fatigued, and any one of these conditions could exist. Other contributing factors also add to the overall stress we perceive, including our work or school schedule with its stressors, home stress, and excessive use of alcohol, drugs, or just a busy social life.

The initial response of many when they experience declining performance in their endurance sport is to train harder. Although this may work in some instances, such as for those who are actually undertraining, this will actually make things worse for those who have been overtraining.

When you experience severe fatigue or declining performance, it is reasonable to consider a short period (1–2 weeks) of relative rest by stepping away from your activity or cross-training while reviewing your nutrition and hydration as well as sleep and other stressors. If you do not recover, you should consider evaluation with a doctor familiar with sports-related overtraining.

Other symptoms that should prompt more urgent evaluation with your doctor would include fever, sweating at night, unintentional weight loss, an unresolving cough, diarrhea lasting more than 1 week, or diarrhea with blood.

16. What are the most commonly missed (misdiagnosed) sports injuries?

When a patient sees a healthcare provider, the patient's greatest liability is the provider. His or her ability to gather the appropriate history, perform an appropriate examination, and understand the list of possibilities (what we call the differential diagnosis) affects a provider's ability to come to an appropriate diagnosis and formulate a plan.

Missed diagnoses may center on all these aspects of a complete office visit. Important components of a differential diagnosis are the patient's providing a good history or story of the complaint and the provider's knowledge of the problems and how to evaluate it. Some diagnoses are not obvious on the first or even second visit, and follow-up evaluation is often necessary before the proper diagnosis is made.

Sports diagnoses that are missed are often very difficult. The most common is a medical problem presenting as a sports-related problem, e.g., fatigue thought to be overtraining but that is related to cancer or anemia, back pain that is actually related to an abdominal aneurysm and shoulder pain that is related to an upper lung tumor. Although rare, these occur in everyday practice.

Less worrisome diagnoses include lower leg blood flow issues called **ischemia**, groin problems, and nerve entrapments, which top the list of missed issues in sports. Many of the specifics in the musculoskeletal diagnoses are covered in the various questions in this book.

Ischemia
Lack of blood flow.

Missed diagnoses of the arm and shoulder such as thoracic outlet syndrome, a nerve and **vascular** pinching in the shoulder causing arm pain; nerve entrapments of various nerves in the arm; and compartment syndrome in the forearm after crushing injuries should be considered.

Vascular
Pertaining to blood flow.

Common misdiagnoses in the abdomen and groin include all the groin issues discussed in Questions 57 and 58, as well as pelvic or hip stress fractures and nerve entrapments.

In the lower extremity, the focus on missed problems would be unusual presentations of stress fractures, nerve impingements from the back or nerve damage in the leg, vascular compromise from pinched vessels called claudication, or even popliteal artery entrapment. Another cause of leg pain is the exertional compartment syndrome. This is covered well in Question 71. Pain in the extremities can also be caused by reflex sympathetic dystrophy (RSD) or what is now known as complex regional pain syndrome (CRPS), which is a pain syndrome often following injury or surgery manifested by severe burning pain, temperature and color changes, and swelling of the affected appendage (hand, foot, leg, or arm).

17. What fractures are unique to children?

Fracture

Broken bone or tooth.

Fractures are a common and unfortunate part of all the play and organized activities in which children participate. Kids often fall and injure a body part with very short-duration pain, and then without any residual symptoms return to play. It is often baffling to parents. Indications of more significant injury would include deformity, swelling, and persistent disuse and splinting of the injured joint or limb. Because the pliability and strength of the bone and the presence of growth plates, there are some fractures that are unique. These are the torus or buckle fracture and the classification of growth plate injuries called **Salter Harris fractures**.

Salter Harris fracture

A classification system for growth plate fractures in children grading them from 1 through 5 in ascending order of severity.

Torus or buckle fractures may occur in any bone but are most commonly seen in the wrist—specifically the radius, the larger bone on the thumb side of the wrist. With some injuries, often those caused by falls, if there is a lower energy impact or deforming stress imparted on the bone, a partial break might occur. Sometimes called the greenstick fracture, this is unique in that rather than both sides of the bone being broken, only one side is broken. On X-ray, it looks like a very subtle buckle. These minor fractures heal very rapidly and may be treated with a cast or even a splint for 2–3 weeks.

The Salter Harris classification was established to define injuries and fractures involving the growth centers. Growth centers, or physes, often exist at each end of a bone to allow lengthening as children grow. These close in a very predictable pattern in adolescence. In children, these growth centers and bone are weak, but there are very strong ligaments. Often an injury that may cause a typical fracture or ligament sprain in an adult will cause a growth plate injury in children. The symptoms are the same as for any other fracture with an injury causing pain, swelling, and inability to use the limb. A classification scale of one through five is used, with the severity of injury increasing with the classification number. It is not important to review the specific classification, but rather the risks. Severe, untreated injuries to the growth centers can cause arrest of the growth plate totally or in one portion or a bony bridge in the middle of a growth center. With this there can be growth cessation and therefore a short limb or curving due to the tethering of the bone bridge and continued growth in the remainder of the growth plate.

18. What causes back pain in kids and how should it be evaluated and managed?

First it should be noted that back pain is not a normal part of life for children and adolescents as it is in adults. Back pain should be taken seriously, especially if associated with functional limitation, as in limping or desire to not participate in activities of play or sport. Back pain requiring more urgent evaluation is that associated with fever or sweats especially at night, weakness in the legs, and bladder function changes, weight loss, or pain at night.

Common diagnoses associated with back pain in children include overuse low back pain, herniated disk, diskitis (infection), **spondylolysis,** and **spondylolisthesis.**

Disk-type pain symptoms are similar to those of adults. Often the pain is not in the back, but rather the buttocks or leg. The pain is usually in the back of the leg aggravated by sitting, coughing, or sneezing. When pain is present with these

Spondylolysis

A fracture of the pars interarticularis of the vertebral body; usually a stress fracture; spondylolysis on both sides at the same level may result in slippage (spondylolisthesis).

Spondylolisthesis

A slippage of one vertebral body on another, usually in the lower back and associated with spondylolysis.

maneuvers, the pain usually shoots down the leg below the knee. It may be associated with difficulty urinating, numbness, or weakness in one or both of the legs.

Diskitis

Infection of the intervertebral disc

Diskitis is an infection of the disk from a bacterial infection. Often children or adolescents afflicted with diskitis will have fever and localized back pain aggravated by direct pressure. They may also have other medical problems like a previous surgery, sickle cell disease, or a prior acute illness.

Spondylolysis and spondylolisthesis are two diagnoses unique to adolescents. In the spine at each vertebral level there is a bridge of bone called the pars interarticularis between the upper and lower facet joints. Facet joints are paired upper and lower joints toward the back and sides at each vertebral level. They articulate with the facet joints of the vertebrae above and below providing further stability. People with spondylolysis will notice pain with impact activity (running and jumping) and with back extension (leaning back). This is often seen in gymnasts, dancers, football linemen, and runners, but it may be seen in any athlete active in an impact activity with extension. The pain is usually one sided and in the back only. Occasionally this is associated with disk-type radiating symptoms, but this is not common. Early on the pain will only be with activity, but as symptoms progress, the child may have pain with simple activities of daily living.

Generally the victim must go through the stress fracture (spondylolysis) stage to get to the slippage of a spondylolisthesis.

Spondylolysis is an overuse stress fracture in the lower back. If this stress fracture progresses and is on both sides at the same spinal level, the child may develop a forward slippage of one vertebra on another called spondylolisthesis. Generally the athlete must go through the stress fracture (spondylolysis) stage to get to the slippage of a spondylolisthesis.

Spondylolysis should be evaluated with a provider familiar with back pain in children. On exam the child will have no pain with forward bending, but will have aggravation of pain when leaning back, especially when leaning back while standing on the left or right leg. Additionally, the child will have tight hip flexors (front of hip) and hamstrings. Evaluations should start with plain X-rays but usually require advanced imaging. This imaging may include bone scan or magnetic resonance imaging (MRI). Bone scan is usually the first advanced study; an MRI is reserved for symptomatic children with strong suspicion for this problem indicated by normal X-rays and bone scan.

Treatment is usually rest from the offending impact activity and avoiding back extension. While doing this, the patient can work on core strengthening and stretching of the hamstrings and hip flexors. This rest may last for 4–12 weeks. In more severe cases, bracing may be recommended, but rarely surgery.

19. What is apophysitis and what does it mean in children?

Apophysitis refers to a common group of overuse diagnoses in children. An apophysis is a secondary growth center at the attachment site of major tendons in the body. These growth centers are not involved in bone longitudinal growth, but only the maturation of this important muscular attachment. Important apophyses are located in the knee, heel, inside elbow, crest of the hip and the ischium in the gluteal area. The underlying theme for all the following diagnoses is overuse. Too much running, throwing, jumping, and tightness in young athletes with growing muscles sets them up for these problems.

Apophysitis
Inflammation of the apophysis in growing athletes.

In the knee the two diagnoses are Osgood-Schlatter disease and Sinding-Larsen-Johansson (SLJ) syndrome. These both refer to inflammation at either end of the patellar tendon that goes from the kneecap to the tibia. Osgood-Schlatter disease refers to inflammation of the attachment of the tendon on the tibia below the knee, and SLJ causes inflammation at the lower pole of the tendon. These are more common in the 12–15-year period. Children may complain of swelling and pain with jumping or running. They may even have a limp. The symptomatic bump will be painful to the touch or kneeling. Treatment of this condition should include ice and ibuprofen or children's ibuprofen in the appropriate dose and relative rest. The inflammation will respond to slowing down for a few days and then the child can return to activity. Often the child will develop pain within a few weeks if the level of activity is not modified. Children will continue to be symptomatic until this growth center has matured, which may take 2 years. One option then is to limit the total amount of impact as in limited practicing to save them for games as well as to work aggressively on hamstring and quadriceps stretching exercises. Additionally, children with Osgood-Schlatter disease may consider wearing a patellar tendon counterforce brace such as the Cho-Pat brace (www.cho-pat.com) for activity.

This same condition of the heel is called Sever's disease. The age onset is usually younger—in the 8–11-year range—and will often be associated with tight calf muscles. Management is similar to that of Osgood-Schlatter disease, although there are not great braces to be worn.

Iliac apophysitis refers to pain at the outside part of the pelvic bone seen in adolescent runners. The pain occurs with running only. This is not too dissimilar to the traumatic hip pointer seen in football and soccer players, but this is an overuse condition. These runners need to work aggressively on iliotibial band stretching and side leg lifts. See Question 60.

Ischium

The pelvic bone in the buttocks or bottom that is the upper attachment site for the hamstring muscle.

The portion of the pelvic bone that we sit on is the origin (beginning) of the hamstring. One can find the **ischium** by bringing the knee to the chest and pushing directly behind the thigh where the thigh joins the buttocks. This apophysis is usually injured by hamstring strain-type injuries rather than overuse. The adolescent will have tight hamstrings associated with sprinting. This should be evaluated by a physician or athletic trainer.

Apophysis on the inside of the elbow is associated with Little League elbow and is further discussed in Question 78.

20. Is weight lifting safe for children?

Resistance (strength) training is safe for children as young as 8–10 years of age. There are many considerations prior to the institution of a weight-training program for young athletes.

The equipment used should be of the proper size and have low enough weights for use by young athletes. There should be adequate lighting. Children should be mature enough to follow instructions and must be supervised at all times. The strength program should be a part of an overall comprehensive program to increase motor skills and fitness.

Training should be 2–3 times per week with single or multi-set programs of 8–15 repetitions. All programs should begin with no weight until the young athlete demonstrates proper form. Weights should be increased in 1–3-pound increments when 15 repetitions are done with proper form. Overhead lifts while standing should be substituted with seated press to minimize **lumbar spine** stresses. No single maximum lift should ever be attempted by young athletes.

Exercises should be carried through the full range of motion of the joint with emphasis on proper breathing. Additionally, there should be a warm-up and warm-down period emphasizing stretching. Young athletes should concentrate on concentric-type programs and leave heavy eccentric training for adults. Concentric exercises involve contraction of a muscle as it is shortening. Eccentric exercises involve contraction of a muscle as it lengthens, i.e., negatives. Eccentric training is much more stressful to muscles and tendons and should be avoided by young athletes.

Although resistance training is effective in preventing many sport-related injuries, certain positions with weight training

Lumbar spine

The lower back, consisting of five vertebrae.

programs can do more harm than good for the shoulder. As a general rule, absolute intensity single-repetition maximum (1 RM) weight lifting should be avoided. A youth who attempts them should limit attempts to two to three times per year.

Abduction

Joint motion moving away from the midline.

Dislocation

Out of place; pertaining to a joint.

Subluxation

Partial dislocation; this may be transient or a joint or tendon may be stuck in this partially dislocated position.

Overhand grip for bench press with hand spacing 1.5 to 2 times the shoulder width is generally recommended. All bench press activities should have a mandatory hand-off when complete. The position of full **abduction** and external rotation of the shoulder that occurs with placing a weight into the cradle after bench press places the shoulder at maximum risk for anterior **dislocation** or **subluxation** (partial dislocation). Inclined bench press should be avoided. A behind-the-neck shoulder press as well as a latissimus pull-down should be avoided. Instead, the latissimus dorsi can be exercised by pulling the bar in front of the neck.

Finally, no competition should be encouraged or allowed. Most injuries to young athletes associated with weight lifting involve competing and lack of adult supervision.

PART TWO

Head, Face, and Neck Injuries

What is a concussion and what should I do about it?

What do I do about nosebleeds?

What should I do about my neck sprain or strain (whiplash injury)?

More . . .

21. What is a concussion and what should I do about it?

A concussion is a temporary impairment of how the brain works due to a force applied to the brain. Concussions come on all of the sudden due to either a direct blow to the head, face, or neck, or an impulse force that travels to the head from somewhere else in the body. The main problem from concussions is how the brain works, not with how healthy the brain is physically; it is a functional problem rather than a structural one. Because of this, certain imaging tests—like head CT (CAT scans), MRI, and X-rays—are usually completely normal in concussions. Symptoms of a concussion may occur suddenly or several hours after the injury. The functional problems in the brain may affect how well you think, feel, behave, speak, and understand things. This resolves with complete rest. Once you start to recover from a concussion, some of the symptoms might change and may even last several months before improving (this is known as postconcussive syndrome). Although it is controversial, world experts in sports concussions agree that fainting or passing out (loss of consciousness), although dramatic and concerning, is not as important as amnesia in the evaluation of severity.

Symptoms of a concussion may occur suddenly or several hours after the injury.

Some of the signs and symptoms suggesting a concussion include:

1. Vacant or glassy-eyed stare
2. Confusion (altered level of consciousness)
3. Inappropriate playing behavior, such as repeatedly executing the wrong play or going to the wrong huddle)
4. Feeling slow, dinged, foggy, dazed, or stunned
5. Slowly answering questions or following commands
6. Distraction and trouble concentrating
7. Trouble remembering things (amnesia)
8. Passing out or fainting (loss of consciousness)
9. Constantly feeling tired or worn out (fatigue)
10. Irritability

11. Emotional, mood, or personality changes
12. Headache/head pressure
13. Balance problems
14. Nausea and vomiting
15. Problems or changes in how the victim sees or hears things
16. Trouble speaking or slurred speech
17. Convulsions, twitching, or shaking of the body while unconscious

These symptoms tend to be worse with physical or mental activity. Although the issue is controversial, symptoms that may be more concerning of a more severe concussion include symptoms with exertion, convulsions, loss of consciousness, a concussion resulting from lesser impact, and a history of multiple concussions over time.

Initial treatment includes basic first aid and deciding whether the athlete needs to go to the hospital or emergency department. If possible, alert a physician, athletic trainer, or other healthcare professional familiar with sports medicine present at the sporting event. Once an athlete is suspected to have a concussion, he or she should be restricted from playing or practice that day, until he or she can be evaluated by a healthcare professional. If you suspect an athlete of having a concussion, consider calling 911 (alerting the emergency medical service) if he or she has:

1. Neck pain
2. Lost consciousness lasting >30 seconds
3. Seizures or convulsions
4. Numbness or tingling in both hands or both feet
5. Lost the ability to move both hands and feet
6. A difference in the size of the pupils
7. Severe and worsening nausea and vomiting
8. Bruising around both eyes or behind both ears
9. Blood or clear fluid leaking from the ears
10. Sudden, profuse, watery runny nose

Initial and follow-up treatment of concussions is best taken care of by a healthcare professional, such as a physician or athletic trainer. In general, a thorough evaluation of the athlete's ability to perform mental exercises and a physical examination are performed. In the hours that follow the injury, the athlete should not be left alone. At some point during the treatment of a concussion, a physician or physician-appointed professional should be involved in caring for the athlete. Usually, the treatment includes ruling out more severe injuries or complications, further testing, and a prescribed rest from physical activity and/or high mental concentration demands. Once the athlete is completely without symptoms at rest, he or she may then start a gradual progression of activity, supervised by a healthcare professional, before a physician or physician-appointed professional clears the athlete to return to sports participation. In some athletes, there may be residual symptoms for several months, called postconcussive syndrome. It has also been theorized that the effects of a concussion may last much longer than previously thought, and there may even be permanent effects. Most people who suffer a concussion, however, do recover.

Currently, there is no research data that support the use of currently available protective equipment to prevent concussions. Protective devices that have been studied include helmets, forehead pads, mouthpieces, and face shields. Protective equipment may prevent other forms of head injury that may be an important consideration for athletes participating in those sports, but the equipment might not protect against concussions, specifically. In general, most athletes are advised to wear the protective equipment that they or their parents feel is necessary to protect them from injury.

22. What should I do about headaches?

As athletes may suffer from the same headache types as the general population, headaches in athletes may be secondary to many causes. Any headache associated with confusion, dizziness, numbness, weakness, tingling, nausea, vision changes, neck stiffness or other nervous system changes may be a sign of a serious condition, and should be evaluated by a physician prior to further athletic participation.

Athletes who have had concussions (see Question 21) may have a headache immediately afterwards, but also during subsequent bouts of exercise, until they have fully recovered from their concussion. For this reason, if your headache began with trauma to the head and neck, you should see your physician for guidelines regarding when and how to return to activity.

Headaches during exercise may also be caused by dehydration and heat-related illness. Adequate hydration is a primary concern during exercise, and athletes should be careful to take in enough fluids. Following urine output is the simplest way to gauge hydration, and urination should be frequent, with clear, rather than dark urine. When exercising in a warm environment, onset of a headache should cue an athlete to pause, rest, and assess his hydration status and temperature.

Migraine headache may be brought on by severe exertion or, in contact sports, trauma. They are typically characterized by unilateral pain, and are often described as throbbing. Visual changes may precede headache onset, and headache may last hours to days. A family history of migraine may or may not be present. Exertional migraines may be associated with and likely share the same mechanism as orgasmic migraines. Orgasmic migraines are more common in men than women. They may begin with arousal, become most severe at orgasm, and usually resolve fairly rapidly. Any severe headache brought on by trauma should be evaluated by a physician. Exertion-induced migraine may be treated with naproxen, ibuprofen, or acetaminophen, or classical migraine drugs such as triptans (Sumatriptan, Tizatriptan, Zolmitriptan, Eletriptan, Naratriptan, etc.). A slow warm-up period may help to prevent exertion migraine. For those with recurrent exertion migraines that

Migraine Headache

Identifies a classification of a headache characterized by acute onset of a throbbing one-sided headache associated with nausea, light sensitivity and occasionally tearing and nasal congestion.

37

are not adequately controlled by the above means, a physician may recommend a daily medicine to decrease the frequency and possibly the duration and severity of the headaches. These medicines are referred to as prophylactic (preventive) medications, and they include calcium channel blockers (Verapamil), beta blockers (Propranolol), topiramate, neurontin, tricyclic antidepressants (Nortriptyline or Amitriptyline), and valproic acid. A straining or weight-lifting headache typically occurs in athletes who strain against a closed airway, or **valsalva**. This is perhaps most common in weight lifting. These headaches are often described as **posterior**, or occipital (in the back of the head), may last for days or longer, and resolve slowly. One explanation for these headaches is that the aforementioned straining increases pressure within the brain. Although they are often benign, these headaches may be secondary to structural disease and should be evaluated by a physician.

Athletes with recurrent headaches during exercise, especially those with a family history of sudden death, brain aneurysm, or polycystic kidneys should be evaluated by their physician for a high blood pressure response to exercise and structural brain disease such as aneurysm.

23. What do I do about nosebleeds?

Nosebleeds are common both in athletes and nonathletes, and they commonly occur in association with cold, dry weather, nose picking, and trauma. Most nosebleeds can be controlled at home without seeing a physician. To control a nosebleed, you should tilt your head and lean forward to keep blood from draining down the back of the throat to be swallowed or interfere with breathing. Direct pressure should be applied to both sides of the distal (near the tip), soft portion of the nose for at least 5 minutes by your watch. If the nose is still bleeding after 5 minutes of direct pressure, pressure should be applied to the nose for another 10 minutes before checking for further bleeding. Ice applied to the firm, upper portion of the nose may be helpful in controlling a nosebleed. If, after

Valsalva

The act of increasing the pressure in the abdomen or chest as when coughing, straining to have a bowel movement, or lifting an object without breathing.

Posterior

Behind or toward the back.

20–30 minutes, your nosebleed has not subsided, you should be evaluated by a physician or visit the emergency room for further intervention.

Recurrent nosebleeds frequently arise from a portion of the nose that can easily be treated by your physician to prevent or decrease further bleeding. If your nosebleed occurs as a result of trauma to the nose, you should see a physician if you have significant deformity, severe pain, or difficulty breathing through your nose. A septal hematoma, or collection of blood beneath the mucosa of the wall of the nasal septum, may appear to you as a severe bruise or blood blister. This should be evaluated by a physician, as it is likely to become infected or cause necrosis of the septum. You should also seek medical attention if you notice other easy bruising or bleeding, such as excessive bleeding with tooth brushing, blood in your urine or stool, or a family history of bleeding disorder.

24. What should I do about facial injuries?

Facial injuries may be divided into lacerations or cuts, blunt trauma to the face, and penetrating, or stab injuries. Any facial laceration that leads to significant bleeding that is not controlled by brief, simple pressure, or is not obviously quite superficial, would likely benefit from evaluation by a physician for suture placement to avoid infection and unnecessary scarring. Any injury that breaks the skin requires thorough cleaning to avoid infection. Debris should be removed, the wound irrigated (flushed with clean water), and then the wound should be cleaned with peroxide or soap and water. Penetrating or stab injuries should also be evaluated by a physician for thorough cleaning and evaluation for damage to underlying structures.

Blunt trauma to the face raises concern for facial fracture and may cause damage to the eye (see Question 25) or an open communication with the central nervous system. You should seek attention for severe pain, loss of consciousness,

If your nosebleed occurs as a result of trauma to the nose, you should see a physician if you have significant deformity, severe pain, or difficulty breathing through your nose.

change in sensation of the face, asymmetry in the appearance or palpation of the face, blurry or double vision, inability to bring your teeth together, change in hearing, or clear discharge from the nose or ear.

25. What should I do about eye injuries?

Most sports-related eye injuries involve blunt trauma. Racket sports such as tennis and racquetball, baseball, and hockey are quite high risk. Basketball, wrestling, and boxing are also thought to involve increased risk to the eye relative to other sports. Other types of eye injuries include penetrating injuries, superficial foreign objects or corneal abrasions, and radiation injuries from sunlight.

Common injuries from blunt trauma include a simple hematoma—or black eye, fracture of the orbital bone, retinal detachment, and fracture of the eye itself, or globe fracture. If you experience blunt trauma to the eye, you should seek medical attention immediately if you experience any of the following: extreme pain; vision changes; sudden onset of multiple, small objects that appear to float across your field of vision known as floaters or flashing lights; double vision; an eye that bulges or appears sunken; numbness around the eye; pain with opening the mouth, irregularly shaped pupil; difficulty moving the eye in any direction; the appearance of blood collecting in the eye; or any damage to the eyeball itself.

All lacerations to the eye require immediate evaluation by a physician. Lacerations of the eyelid require evaluation for full complete penetration of the lid and subsequent damage to the underlying globe. Penetrating foreign objects, e.g., glass, plant life, etc., should not be removed on site, but prevented from moving and causing more damage and evaluated immediately in the emergency department. Foreign body sensation in the eye should also always be evaluated by a physician, as should the appearance of blood in the eye.

Radiation injuries most commonly occur when engaging in water sports or in a snowy environment. Care should be taken in these settings to protect the eyes from UV light with appropriate eyewear. Symptoms may include redness, pain, and increased pain when exposed to bright light.

26. What should I do about jaw injuries?

Similar to facial injuries, jaw injuries are not uncommon in sports involving hard contact with little facial protection, such as hockey, skiing, boxing, wrestling, rugby, and field hockey. At initial evaluation of such injuries, one must first assess if there has been any neck injury or whether the individual has sustained a concussion. These issues are covered well in Questions 21 and 29. Dental injuries are also covered in Question 28. Jaw injuries may run the gamut from bruises and soft tissue injury to lacerations and fractures. Bleeding should be stopped with direct pressure, and if the wound is deep, the bleeding cannot be stopped, or there is any question about the management, the individual should be transported to the emergency room.

Fractures of the jaw (mandible) may be manifested by deformity, pain, and crunching over the fractured area. **Malocclusion** (abnormal alignment of the teeth when attempting to bite), inability chew, or excessively painful chewing in the absence of a tooth injury are all concerning symptoms for jaw fracture. Occasionally a milder injury to the TMJ joint after such injury may result in clicking of the TMJ with a persistent more mild pain long after the injury.

Malocclusion
Abnormal alignment of teeth.

The most important thing about these injuries is that bleeding and swelling may interfere with the ability to breathe, and if there is concern that this might occur, someone should call EMS. Otherwise, individuals with any of the above worsening signs of injury should be evaluated in the emergency room and likely will need advanced imaging and evaluation by a maxillofacial specialist or plastic surgeon.

27. How should I treat cauliflower ear?

Cauliflower ear is a term used for injuries to the ear from wrestling, rugby, and boxing, although any activity with repetitive blows or friction on the ear may cause similar problems. With repeated friction or direct blows, a blood clot forms between the cartilage and skin of the ear. With initial injury this clot is soft and very painful. Individuals with cauliflower ear will have pain with any manipulation of the ear and even with talking or chewing. Initial treatment may include pain medications like ibuprofen, naproxen, or acetaminophen and application of ice to minimize further bleeding and to treat pain.

Your doctor may drain this acute clot or make an incision to drain it. After a few days, the initial bleeding may harden and aspiration will not be possible for 7–10 days until the clot starts to soften, favoring incision as the treatment in these cases.

After drainage, some type of pressure device should be applied. These are quite difficult to apply and keep in place, especially if the individual is still going to participate in sports. Such pressure options include gauze dressings inside and behind the ear and an elastic wrap around the head. Another option is gauze material soaked in collodian (a very odd-smelling fluid that will cause the gauze to harden). This may be placed inside the ear to maintain the shape. Finally, doctors may suture a pressure dressing on the ear. If nothing is done, the clot will become less painful over a 2- to 3-week period and harden, forming a scar. Such scarring will deform the ear and reduce its ability to trap sound. At this point, the only option to fix the ear is surgery by a plastic surgeon or Otolaryngologist (Ear Nose and Throat doctor). This latter option is only suggested when an athlete has reached the end of his or her sports career and is not likely to receive further blows to the ear.

Prevention is the best strategy. Wearing headgear at all times when wrestling, boxing, or playing the scrum position in rugby is the best prevention. This includes games and practices. As in many similar problems, most of the injuries occur in practice.

28. What should I do about loose, broken, or knocked-out teeth?

Dental injuries may occur as an isolated injury or in combination with other facial and jaw injuries. When there is a concern for such injuries the simplest test is to run your tongue over your teeth to detect any defects not noted before. Open the jaw and attempt to chew. Isolated pain may be an indication of a facial or jaw fracture or dental injury.

Traumatic tooth injuries include loosened teeth (**luxation**, **extrusion**, and intrusion), broken teeth (fracture), and complete removal of a tooth from the socket (avulsion). These are considered dental urgencies or emergencies, which mean you should be evaluated by a dental or healthcare provider and perhaps have an X-ray as soon as possible. Some complications of more significant injuries include infection, death of the tooth, loss of the tooth, and other associated mouth and facial injuries.

Broken teeth (fractured teeth) are usually obvious (broken outside the gum line), but can also be less obvious (inside the gums). You may need to get an X-ray to find fractures inside the gums. The inside contents of the tooth (pulp) may leak from a fracture. This is typically very painful and should be evaluated by a dentist sooner rather than later. Any part of the tooth that broke off (tooth fragment) should be kept wet and hydrated, since the dentist may be able to reattach it. Wrap any broken parts and the remnants of the broken tooth with a moist cotton ball and see your dentist. The injured tooth may also need a root canal treatment or even be pulled out (extraction) if the injury is severe enough.

Teeth can be loosened in different directions. In general, these should be ultimately treated by a dentist who may need to

Luxation

A term for partial dislocation; aka, subluxation; a term applied to partially dislocated teeth

Extrusion

Tooth movement in the direction of eruption

Any part of the tooth that broke off (tooth fragment) should be kept wet and hydrated, since the dentist may be able to reattach it.

reposition or splint the tooth, perform a root canal treatment, or even pull the tooth (extraction). Avoid chewing or using the injured teeth, and seek professional attention. You may need antibiotics and possibly a tetanus shot if you haven't had one in the last 5 years.

If a tooth has been completely pulled or knocked out of the socket by the injury (avulsion), it is important to retrieve and protect the avulsed tooth, so the dentist can possibly reimplant it into the socket. If possible, simply put the tooth back into the socket immediately after the injury. If dirty, the tooth can be gently rinsed in cold water before placing it into the socket. Do not let anything touch, rub, or hit the root of the tooth (the part that goes into the socket). If you cannot put the tooth back into the socket, put the tooth in the mouth, between the gum and inside of the cheek. You could also put the tooth in milk. You should then see a dentist as soon as possible. You will also need antibiotics, and possibly a tetanus shot if you haven't had one in the last 5 years.

To prevent these dental and other injuries, appropriately fitted mouth guards and face shields should be used in participation in sports. While custom-fitted mouthpieces can be obtained from your dental care professional, most commercially available mouthpieces are good enough.

29. What should I do about my neck sprain or strain (whiplash injury)?

Sprain

Injury of a muscle; graded 1–3.

Strain

Injury to a ligament; graded 1–3.

Flexion

Joint motion in which the joint moves closer to the body.

Neck injuries include several diagnoses. These include broken bones (fracture), stretched or torn ligaments (**sprains**), muscle and tendon injuries (**strains**), herniated disks, and injuries to other structures like nerves, blood vessels, and the throat (both the airways used for breathing and the esophagus used for swallowing). Most injuries involve the muscles, tendons, ligaments, and bones. Many of these injuries are caused by the whiplash mechanism, in which the neck is quickly thrown into a forced **flexion** (bending forward, chin towards chest) or extension (bending head back, chin away from chest) position. This can cause ligaments to sprain and muscles to strain, leading to muscle spasms that can be very painful, and which stiffen the neck muscles, limiting range of motion. Usually, this pain and stiffness is limited to the areas in the back and sides of the neck, on either side of the midline. If you have symptoms in the midline of the neck, this may be more significant than just a sprain or strain. If you have symptoms of neck injury other than a mild to moderate sprain or strain, you should consult your healthcare professional (see Question 30). Otherwise you can try the following home treatment and rehabilitation exercises, and see how you do:

1. *Relative rest*—Avoiding quick and painful movements in the neck initially after the injury can be helpful, but it is important to limit this rest to the first 1–2 weeks after the injury. As soon as comfortable, you should try to use your neck as you normally would.

2. *Ice versus heat*—Ice used following the injury can help with pain relief (see Question 10), but muscle spasm can set in, leading to stiffness and a tight, achy pain in the areas around the spine. Heat, such as a warm heating pad, can be very useful in alleviating spasm. Basically, start with ice, then move to heat in 1–2 days. Try both, and whichever one helps is the one you should use.

3. *Massage*—Massaging also helps alleviate muscle spasm.

4. *Stretching and strengthening*—Stretching and strengthening exercises should initially be used gently, and then increased as your neck recovers. This speeds healing, alleviates spasm, and helps prevent further injury. (see **Figure 1** on page 169)

5. *Medications*—Various over-the-counter medications may be helpful as well (see Question 11).

Most neck injuries will respond to this self-treatment within 1–2 weeks. Recovery should progress nicely within 2–4 weeks. If you find that your symptoms are worsening or not improving after 3–4 weeks, consult your healthcare professional. Incidentally, long-term, more chronic cases of neck pain are closely associated with poor workplace ergonomics and the head-forward, rounded shoulder posture.

Prevention of sports-related neck injuries includes training exercises focused on the flexibility, endurance, and strengthening of the muscles that support the neck. These exercises should themselves be introduced gradually and include neck movements in all directions of motion, even if the actual sporting activity only calls for one or two directions of neck motion. In addition to providing a more comprehensive prevention program, doing so also prevents an overuse injury.

Overuse injuries are common in the neck. This occurs when one uses the neck, in the same way, over and over again. This repetitive motion can lead to inflammation, swelling, pain, and even small microscopic tears in tendons, muscles, and ligaments. This is especially common in the workplace, especially in this age of computers and workstations, where people might maintain the same posture, or repeat the same motions all day long. These overuse injuries can be very difficult to treat, and may even become a chronic condition.

The mainstay to treating chronic, overuse injuries is to initially stop the offending activity, rest, rehabilitate, gradually reintroduce the activity, and prevent reinjury. It is important to include strategies to avoid repeating the same motions over and over again. This may include frequent breaks, stretching during the activity, and observing correct ergonomics. For example, prolonged sitting at a workstation tends to promote a head-forward, rounded-shoulder, and forward-leaning posture that puts a continuous stress on the muscles and ligaments in the back of the neck. This, in turn, may lead to an overuse injury of the neck. Taking the time to stretch and perform some of the neck rehabilitation exercises, however, may help prevent this from occurring in the first place.

Many of the same treatment options used for acute neck injuries may also be useful for chronic overuse injuries. However, treating overuse injuries generally requires more involved rehabilitation exercises and perhaps more sophisticated ways to control pain and stiffness. This may include physical or occupational therapy, massage, and prescription medications. Certain injections into problematic muscles may also be helpful in these cases. See your healthcare provider if you think you may benefit from these treatment options. Again, the best way to treat overuse injuries is to prevent them.

30. When should I see a doctor about my neck pain?

While many neck problems can improve and resolve on their own (see Questions 29 and 31), there are some warning signs that warrant an evaluation and further treatment from a physician or healthcare provider. They include:

1. Midline neck pain (pain in the middle of the neck, as opposed on either side of the spine).
2. Numbness, tingling, profound muscle weakness in both left and right arms, forearms, and hands.
3. Severe worsening of your neck pain with neck movement, especially minor motion to the neck.
4. Trouble breathing, talking, swallowing, or signs of injuries to anything other than muscles, tendons, and ligaments (this may even warrant emergency evaluation).
5. Symptoms of a concussion (see Question 21).
6. Loss of consciousness (this may be a more urgent problem).
7. Neck symptoms fail to improve within an expected period of time (see Questions 29 and 31).
8. Discomfort with self-treatment.

Your physician or other healthcare provider will want to obtain details of how you were injured and perform an examination of your neck and upper extremities. He or she may order X-rays of the neck from several different angles or in various positions. If any position is much too painful, alert the professional taking the X-ray. Other tests may be ordered by your healthcare provider as well.

31. What is a burner (stinger)? What should I do about it?

A burner or a stinger is a common injury in many sports, including football, soccer, hockey, rugby, wrestling, and lacrosse. It is an injury to a large bundle of nerves (called the brachial plexus) between the spine and the arm, located between the neck and the shoulder. When the neck is quickly thrown in a forced side-tilted position or side-to-side manner, the brachial plexus can be stretched or compressed, injuring the nerves within it. This can lead to numbness, tingling, or a pins-and-needles feeling shooting down the arm, forearm, and hand. There may also be muscle weakness in those areas—including the biceps, supraspinatus, infraspinatus, deltoid, and the hand and wrist flexor muscles. This often shows up as weakness or clumsiness in shoulder movements (especially lifting your arms to the side), bending the elbow, bending and turning the wrist, and especially hand and finger motion and coordination. Often, the shoulder will droop as well.

These are usually mild injuries, however, which resolve with rest from using the neck or that particular arm, and avoiding contact or collision activities. Symptoms usually go away completely within minutes to hours. However, more severe injuries can take days, weeks, or even months to resolve completely. In these cases, you should be seen and followed by a healthcare professional. Persistent weakness may require physical or occupational therapy. Rarely, symptoms fail to completely resolve. Deciding when it is safe to return to play can be a controversial topic, but generally you may return to play once:

- All symptoms have resolved.
- A healthcare professional has examined you and found that you have pain-free, full range of motion of both the neck and the affected upper extremity.
- A healthcare professional has found that you have a normal neurologic examination, paying particular attention to muscle strength.
- You have not had multiple, repeated burners (stingers).

When returning to play, it is very important to do so gradually and with the proper equipment. Shoulder pads, special neck collars (like cowboy collars), and other devices help control the stress applied to the neck and shoulder, protecting the brachial plexus. You may gradually return to noncontact drills and finally to collision or tackle work wearing one of these protective devices.

In general, burners and stingers only affect *one side*. If you have symptoms on both sides or if you have significant neck pain in the midline, you should seek medical attention as soon as possible, since this could represent a spinal cord injury, which can be dangerous.

If you have symptoms on both sides or if you have significant neck pain in the midline, you should seek medical attention as soon as possible, since this could represent a spinal cord injury, which can be dangerous.

PART THREE

Upper Extremity Injuries

What is shoulder impingement or rotator cuff tendonitis, and what should I do about it?

What should I do if my shoulder pops out of socket?

What is a frozen shoulder, and what should I do about it?

More . . .

32. What is shoulder impingement or rotator cuff tendonitis, and what should I do about it?

Rotator cuff

The four stabilizing muscles of the shoulder; these muscles form a continuous tendon over the upper portion of the humerus or arm bone; these muscles are the supraspinatus, infraspinatus, teres minor and subscapularis.

Scapula

The shoulder blade.

Before beginning a discussion about shoulder problems it is best to have a basic discussion of the function of the shoulder and explain what the **rotator cuff** is and what it does. The rotator cuff is a term use to describe four steering muscles deep in the shoulder joint. These four muscles come from the shoulder blade (**scapula**) and attach to the upper arm. The muscles are the supraspinatus, infraspinatus, teres minor and subscapularis, and they are often identified as the SITS muscles. They attach to the upper front to upper back side to the arm in that order (subscapularis-supraspinatus-infraspinatus-teres minor). These muscles form a continuous tendon that cups the upper arm, stabilizing the joint. The shoulder has an unbelievable range of motion that allows us to do all the things we do with it—throw a ball, reach behind us, and reach across and overhead. The upper arm bone (humerus) has a ball joint and the shoulder blade has a small cup for the arm bone to attach to (the glenoid). The best analogy of this relationship is a golf ball on a golf tee. The golf ball easily falls off the tee. There is a glenoid labrum (part of the joint capsule) and ligaments to stabilize this joint, but most of the stability when the shoulder is moving is from the rotator cuff. All our power to do the things we do with our shoulder come from the large muscles we can see and feel, like the pectoralis (chest muscles), deltoid (large muscle directly over the shoulder joint) and the latissimus (back muscle).

Bursa

Potential space that allows tendons, muscles, and skin to slide past each other in a frictionless manner. Can be found throughout the body.

In the event of wear and tear, acute injury, or weakness from disuse and overuse, the rotator cuff does not do its job adequately and the humeral head moves around too much with activity at home, work, or with sports, causing pain. This pain is often called impingement or rotator cuff tendonitis or tendinopathy. With impingement, the rotator cuff and the **bursa** over it become pinched between the acromion (flat bone on top) and the upper humerus (the arm bone or the "golf ball"). Tendinopathy refers to degeneration in the rotator cuff tendon with lack of function and pain with use. This degenerative tendon is painful and has a greater risk for tearing, causing a rotator cuff tear. Rather than a linear tear, tears in the tendon resemble holes. Holes in the tendon can be small with mild pain and weakness or large with significant pain and weakness. The whole diagnosis of impingement, tendonitis, tendinopathy, and tears, rather than individual diagnoses and problems, probably represent more of a continuum of the same process of varying degrees of severity. People with these problems notice shoulder or even upper outside or front arm pain with lifting or reaching overhead and often complain of night pain awakening them.

Typical symptoms are pain in front or the side of the shoulder at night and with recreational and occupational reaching out from the body or overhead. This pain may also be associated with loss of motion. Sometimes it is hard to distinguish between true loss of motion and that associated with pain.

Management of this problem is not an overnight cure. Initial treatment includes ice and pain medications. Avoid reaching away from the body or overhead, especially with any heavy weight in the hand. Exercises to strengthen the rotator cuff in nonpainful positions should be performed as demonstrated in **Figure 2** on page 172. Results with rehabilitation exercises will be slow, and you must be patient.

Consider seeking professional help and evaluation for X-rays if there is a history of an injury or pain lasting more than 1–2 months or not responding to these exercises. Additionally, you may seek a referral to a physical therapist for organized and supervised rehabilitative exercises and use of other pain managing treatments like ultrasound, electric stimulation and others.

Additionally, most patients with rotar cuff dysfunction will benefit from scapular strengthening as demonstrated in Figure 3 on page 173.

Comments from Joyce Pendleton—*For several weeks, I sustained severe pain in my right shoulder. It was extremely difficult*

The whole diagnosis of impingement, tendonitis, tendinopathy, and tears, rather than individual diagnoses and problems, probably represent more of a continuum of the same process of varying degrees of severity.

to raise my arm and do everyday tasks. I was referred to Dr. Howard by my primary care physician. Dr. Howard diagnosed the problem and treated me with an injection and suggested home exercises. As a result of the excellent treatment and daily exercises on my part, my pain has decreased significantly. It is easy to see that if one follows the doctor's advice, the end results are positive. He/she certainly has the expertise to diagnose and prescribe; however, it is the patient's responsibility to subsequently follow through on what is recommended.

33. How should I treat an AC (acromioclavicular) sprain?

The acromioclavicular joint is also called the AC joint. This joint is on top of the shoulder. Injuries to this joint are more commonly known as shoulder separation. People sustain a separation when they fall onto the shoulder with the arm at the side or strike or are struck on top of the shoulder as in tackling or hitting a wall. Such falls may injure the AC joint, cause a clavicle (collar bone) fracture, injure the SC (sterno-clavicular) joint, which is the end of the collar bone in front of the neck, or tear the rotator cuff.

Shoulder separations are always injuries and not overuse problems. When the shoulder is separated there may be tearing of ligaments and other soft tissues and even a fracture (broken bone). For this reason these injuries should usually be x-rayed to ensure there is no broken bone or dislocation. People with old separations and prior overuse may develop arthritis in the AC joint, but that is a different problem.

Someone who suffers such an injury will likely notice swelling and bruising over the top of the shoulder. There may be a deformity consisting of a large bump over the AC joint that is different than the other side. If you have a shoulder separation, you will notice pain in this area with shoulder motions especially if you are trying to reach across to the other shoulder or hold the arm out in front.

Initial treatment should include ice and pain medications like acetaminophen, ibuprofen, or naproxen. A sling may be required to control pain. If there is no broken bone on X-ray, the sling may be used for pain only. As the pain diminishes over the upcoming days or weeks depending on severity, motion exercises should be started. Initially, you should begin with pendulum exercises and as motion and pain improve, add wall climbs (see **Figure 4** on page 174) and then transition into rotator cuff strengthening exercises as discussed in Question 32. This process may take 2–12 weeks depending on the severity of the initial injury.

If you have a separated shoulder, you should avoid contact sports until you have full shoulder motion—you should be able to reach overhead, reach the opposite shoulder, and scratch your back—without pain. You should also be able to do 10 push-ups without pain.

34. What should I do if my shoulder pops out of socket?

Shoulder dislocation or laxity is more common with the younger age group, although it can occur at any age. The shoulder may dislocate in any of three directions—frontward, back, and below, but 85% of the time it is to the front. The motion causing this is usually with the arm elevated to the side 90° and the forearm rotated out as in the throwing position. This can happen with tackling or falling on the shoulder with it in this position.

Shoulder dislocation

An injury that occurs when the top of the arm bone loses contact with the socket of the shoulder blade.

When the shoulder dislocates to the front the head of the humerus becomes trapped in front of the front edge of the glenoid. Besides pain you may note tingling in the fingertips or the side of the shoulder and upper arm. For a first-time dislocation, there should be no attempt to relocate it immediately. You should be transported to an emergency room for X-ray and appropriate management.

If you are in a remote location from medical care or this is a recurrent dislocation, self- or on-field relocation could be attempted. A self-reduction technique involves sitting with the hands clasped in front of the knee. While relaxing the shoulder, push the knee out for 20–25 seconds in an attempt to relocate the joint. The sooner this is attempted, the better to minimized severe muscle spasm that must be overcome to successfully relocate (see **Figure 5** on page 175).

A two-person technique is also demonstrated. You should be supine on the ground with the affected arm raised to the side. The person performing the relocation sits on the ground with one foot firmly applied high in your armpit. Grasping the forearm high up, the person doing the relocation slowly leans back, applying a very slow, constant traction on the arm. The relocation will be identified by a sudden lengthening of the arm, a "clunk," and **reduction** in pain and ability to move it. Attempts to self-reduce or assist a reduction should only be tried once or twice, and if it is unsuccessful, you should be taken to the emergency room.

Reduction

Placing a dislocated joint or broken bone back in place.

Recovery after reduction should include a short period of immobilization with a sling until the pain is reduced. Rotator cuff strengthening should be performed as demonstrated in Question 32. The dislocation positioning of abduction and external rotation (raising your hand) should be avoided while rehabilitating. Visualize that there are four quadrants of space in the front your shoulder, divided by a vertical and horizontal plane through the shoulder. Moving the hand to the inside lower and upper quadrants are the most tolerated. The outside below and especially the upper out quadrants should be avoided to prevent further dislocation.

A similar issue is shoulder laxity. People will complain of the shoulder going out or feeling like it wants to do so when their arm is in certain positions. Usually this sensation will be when they are doing activities with the arm in the upper, outer quadrant as mentioned in the previous paragraph. Management includes avoiding this position if possible, and rotator cuff strengthening as discussed in **Figure 2** on page 172. Some athletes, such as football players, may wear a brace to limit the arm getting into this elevated positioning. This is generally only useful for certain athletes who can wear such a brace for their sport activity like football or rugby as opposed to volleyball or swimming.

Persons with repeated dislocations and/or looseness in the shoulder should consider evaluation by an orthopedic surgeon to consider shoulder stabilization surgery.

35. What is a frozen shoulder, and what should I do about it?

Frozen shoulder, also known as adhesive capsulitis, is a common problem in middle-aged individuals following a long period of immobilization or injury or in diabetics or heart patients for unknown reasons. Referring back to the discussion in Question 32 about the joint capsule, frozen shoulder is a contraction or shrinkage of this capsule.

Often people with a frozen shoulder will notice a rapid or gradual loss of shoulder motion, usually with pain. When you move your arms overhead in front or to the side, you use the glenohumeral joint (shoulder joint) and also cause the shoulder blade to slide to the side and rotate. The first 60° of raising an arm to the side going overhead is almost all at the shoulder joint, and beyond this there is an estimated 2:1 ratio of shoulder motion to movement of the scapula to give a smooth motion.

People with frozen shoulder will notice reduced motion with pain. If they look at themselves in the mirror and attempt to raise the affected arm overhead, they will notice an exaggeration of shoulder blade motion and pinching of the neck because of limited shoulder motion. Additionally, they will notice that they cannot reach behind as if to scratch their back. Similar to impingement (Question 32) they will have pain with reaching and lifting objects and at night.

The natural history of most cases of frozen shoulder is that it will thaw in time, although this may take 12–18 months if it is left alone. The main goal is to return motion to normal and restore strength to the rotator cuff muscles. Most individuals cannot push themselves hard enough to recover rapidly, and evaluation and referral to physical therapy is suggested. Refer to the stretching and range of motion exercises demonstrated in **Figure 6** on page 176. Before stretching, apply a hot, moist towel for 10–15 minutes to soften tissues and make them more pliable.

Early on, pain management and motion take priority.

The major goals are motion and strengthening. Early on, pain management and motion take priority. Exercises should start with pendulum exercises, with short wall climbs and broom handle and towel exercises later. Each session should last 20–30 minutes with motion exercises first and strengthening exercises second. Ice may be applied for pain after the activity is done. If you are in physical therapy, you will do these exercises 2–3 days per week, but ideally you should try to do these most days of the week if you want results. As motion is pushed, there may be occasional popping; it is not uncommon for popping to be followed by a dramatic improvement in motion. Most individuals will remark that their motion is good when they can put the back of their hand flat in the small of their back, even if the motion is not equal to the other shoulder.

36. When should I see a surgeon about my shoulder problem?

You should be evaluated for acute injury or fracture management or when chronic shoulder problems have failed to respond to conservative management with time, medications, and rehabilitative exercises. Acute fractures, shoulder separations, and dislocations should be managed in the emergency room by an orthopedist or trained sports physician.

If you have chronic problems, you should consider orthopedic evaluation given the following general conditions:

1. Frozen shoulder failing to respond to aggressive rehabilitation for 6 months
2. Rotator cuff tear with inability to raise the arm to shoulder level
3. Shoulder impingement/tendonitis failing to respond to aggressive therapy for 6 months
4. Recurrent dislocations despite good rehabilitative exercises
5. First dislocation for younger patients; which indicates a high risk of recurrent dislocation
6. Any injury associated with nerve damage
7. Insurance requirements prior to the approval of MRI

37. What is tennis elbow, and what should I do about it?

Tennis elbow, also known as **lateral** (outside) epicondylitis, is tendonitis of the outside of the elbow. Muscles attaching to the outside of the elbow are the extensors that push the wrist and fingers back. Of the various muscles involved, the most commonly involved is the wrist extensor called the extensor carpi radialis brevis (ECRB). Because the involved muscles cross two joints, the elbow and the wrist, they are most symptomatic if activated while both the wrist and elbow are fully stretched out (extended).

Lateral
Outside or farther from the midline.

People with tennis elbow often do not play tennis. Often the symptoms start as insidious elbow pain with reaching and grabbing activities. This may follow a new strain, home building or gardening project, a new exercise program (such as weight lifting), new equipment (such as a racket) or other occupational and recreational overuse activities. People will complain of pain with grabbing and lifting or even shaking hands. The elbow will be sensitive to direct pressure or if accidentally bumped. There may be local swelling over the bump above and outside the elbow. Often this involves the elbow of the dominant arm.

As with other muscular problems the management includes controlling the pain, stretching and strengthening exercises, bracing, and friction massage. Pain management includes pain medications such as acetaminophen, ibuprofen, naproxen, and narcotic medications. Ice or cold packs are very effective for these problems when applied for 12–15 minutes. The ice may be crushed in a bag or a cube can be used to massage the elbow. The best cold pack application is a bag of frozen peas or corn. The latter is prepackaged, reusable, contains real ice, and is most effective.

Exercises include stretching and strengthening exercises as demonstrated in **Figure 7** on page 177. Stretching should be slow and should be held for 25–30 seconds. Strengthening should be performed slowly for ten repetitions and three sets daily. Weight for these exercises should be 2–4 pounds only.

People with tennis elbow often purchase and use tennis elbow straps but have a misconception of how these help and how to apply them. First, it is important to realize that these straps are equal to a crutch. They cure nothing and only allow those afflicted to be active with less pain while rehabilitating and recovering. Therefore they need to be worn only while symptoms are occurring. They should generally not be used around the house and not to bed, but should be used while exercising or doing manual work. The center of the brace should be over the extensor muscle group of the forearm just below the elbow. The top of the brace should be two fingers below the elbow crease. The brace should be applied snugly and then made tight after making a tight fist. When it is properly applied, it should feel tight when you make a fist but merely snug when the fist is relaxed. There are some recent reports of successful management of tennis elbow with a wrist rather that elbow brace. A simple wrist brace to support wrist extension may significantly reduce pain with activity. Rehabilitative exercises are still needed to recover.

Massage can be a valuable management tool that one can use for this condition. The tendon is degenerated. Stretching and resistance exercise stimulate the tendon to heal itself. This is done by enhancing blood flow and the normal healing process. We can further stimulate this with massage. Apply a moist compress to the outside of the elbow for 10 minutes, then, using the thumb of the opposite hand, massage deeply across the painful tendon for 5 minutes. Ice may be applied for pain relief as well taking the various pain medications mentioned previously. Because this induces local damage and pain friction, massage should only be done every 3 days to allow recovery between sessions.

All the home treatments discussed can be initiated prior to any medical evaluation. Consider evaluation with a physician for any acute injury or severe pain and lack of use. Injections of cortisone are often utilized for tennis elbow, but these generally are only pain-managing strategies that allow you to proceed with rehabilitation. Rehabilitation can also be accomplished under the supervision of a physical therapist.

People with tennis elbow who have a good evaluation and have failed to respond to aggressive therapy for 6 months might consider surgical management of their problems. An orthopedic surgeon can be consulted, but a general orthopedist or a hand surgeon is adequate. Surgery will be followed by a recovery period and then 3–6 months of formal physical therapy.

38. What is golfer's elbow, and what should I do about it?

Golfer's elbow, also known as medial epicondylitis, is tennis elbow of the inner aspect of the elbow. The underlying cause is the same except that the muscles involved are the flexors of the wrist and hand. These are the gripping and wrist flexion muscles.

Golfer's elbow is seen in golfers who are pushing their game, especially if they are practicing and playing a lot, like to draw or hook the ball, and take large divots.

Golfer's elbow is seen in golfers who are pushing their game, especially if they are practicing and playing a lot, like to draw or hook the ball, and take large divots. Like tennis elbow, this diagnosis is not limited to golfers and most people with this problem do not play golf. As with tennis elbow, golfer's elbow often accompanies a report of a new home project, weight-lifting program (especially curls), or any other repetitive lifting activity. Pain will occur with activation of the flexor muscles of the elbow, wrist, and fingers, with local swelling and pain when bumped. Because the ulnar nerve (funny bone) is on the **medial** aspect of the elbow, golfer's elbow may be associated with problems with this nerve. See Question 40 concerning cubital tunnel syndrome.

Medial

Inside or closer to the midline.

The exam is similar to that for tennis elbow except that the painful activities include elbow flexion, wrist flexion, gripping the hand, and pronation (turning the palm down). These symptoms will be worse with testing when the elbow is fully straight and less when it is bent.

The rehabilitation is the same as for tennis elbow. Refer to Question 37 for the recommended program including bracing, stretching, strengthening of the finger flexors (also see **Figure 8** on page 178), and wrist and elbow flexors, massage, and bracing.

39. What is bursitis of the elbow, and how should it be treated?

Bursas are potential fluid spaces that we have throughout the body that allow the skin and tendons to slide past each other and over bony prominences in a frictionless manner. Major bursas exist over the back of the elbow, front of the knee, outside the hip, and the back of the ankle and shoulder.

Bursas become inflamed from multiple causes. Most common is single-event injury; such as falling on the elbow, or repetitive direct pressure. The elbow bursa is called the olecranon bursa, and it may also be inflamed from gout.

When your olecranon bursa is inflamed, you may note swelling behind the elbow; it may or may not be painful, hot, or red. Simple, more common, bursitis is characterized by minimally painful swelling (called "Popeye arm") that is not warm or red. More painful, red, hot swelling should prompt urgent evaluation.

Treatments for olecranon bursitis can range from watchful waiting with naproxen or ibuprofen and a compression wrap to aspiration and steroid injection. There is some belief that repeated aspiration and steroid injection may increase the risk of infection. Warm swelling may be consideration for aspiration to diagnose minor infection, or it should be evaluated for gout.

Reaccumulation and chronic bursitis may be a consideration for surgical consultation for removal of the bursa. This option is rarely indicated.

40. What is cubital tunnel syndrome, and how do I treat it?

Cubital tunnel syndrome is a term used to identify ulnar nerve (the funny bone) problems in and around the elbow.

The ulnar nerve runs down the medial aspect of the upper arm and forearm and provides sensation for the ring and pinky fingers and strength to some of the small muscles in the hand.

The nerve can be injured from a single or chronic injury. Acute injuries occur with falls onto the elbow or certain fractures in which the nerve may be directly crushed or torn. More commonly, people have chronic issues with the nerve caused by resting on the elbow for work, recreation, or flexing the elbow too long. The nerve is very tight in the groove to the back and inside the elbow, and when the elbow is flexed beyond 90 degrees, the stretching of the nerve can cause problems with stretching or slipping out of its groove and snapping over the medial epicondyle (the bony prominence on the inside of the elbow), called subluxation.

Common symptoms include numbness in the last two fingers of the hand or elbow and forearm pain. Often the numbness is at night or when resting on the bent elbow for long periods in one position. Often these symptoms are transient and can be shaken off just by straightening out the arm and shaking the hand or taking the pressure off the elbow. As this chronic nerve injury worsens, symptoms will not resolve with simple arm repositioning.

Treatments can include splints at night to limit bending of the elbow and pressure on the nerve, eliminating prolonged flexion of the elbow beyond 90 degrees. Also, those with cubital tunnel syndrome should avoid resting on the elbow. In more severe cases, there are surgical procedures that can be done to dissect the constricting band or loosen pressure on the nerve. Surgery is rarely performed and is not always the best option.

People with cubital tunnel syndrome should seek medical evaluation for severe pain, weakness with hand grip, or numbness that does not resolve with simple straightening of the elbow and shaking the hand.

41. What should I do about my wrist pain?

Wrist problems, like any other joint complaint, can be broken down in to acute, chronic, and acute on chronic problems. Most acute injuries are from falls and involved the fall onto the outstretched hand (FOOSH), i.e., with the wrist back. With such falls people may sustain a fracture or a sprain. Fractures may include the scaphoid, radius, and/or ulna, or other lesser important bones of the wrist or some dislocations. Indications for acute management and X-rays would be significant or obvious deformity of the wrist with severe swelling, especially if there is numbness in the hand. In the absence of these symptoms it is reasonable to splint the wrist and apply ice, get relative rest, and observe for persistent symptoms or resolution.

Chronic wrist pain with or without an obvious injury, especially pain that limits activity, should be evaluated by a physician. Common diagnoses include missed fracture of the wrist, scapholunate dislocation, triangular fibrocartilage complex (TFCC) injury, arthritis, or tendonitis—most commonly DeQuervain's tenosynovitis. Besides pain with activity, one may also note swelling. Pain on the thumb side of the wrist may indicate a concerning fracture or tendonitis, and pain on the outside (small finger side) may indicate a TFCC problem. Scapholunate dissociation pertains to a tear of the ligaments between these two **carpal bones**. If you have this injury, you will have pain with rotation or pushing off with the hand, as well clicking and swelling with activity. Evaluation of these symptoms should include exam and X-rays and advanced imaging with MRI or bone scan.

Carpal bones
The eight bones in the wrist.

DeQuervain's tendonitis is the most common tendonitis in the wrist. Additionally, it is the most common tendonitis in pregnant women and young mothers. Across the top of the wrist there are six narrow compartments through which all the extensor tendons pass. The first compartment is located in the area of the radial styloid, the bump on the radius (wrist bone) at the base of the thumb. With DeQuervain's, you will notice swelling and pain in this area. You will have pain with attempts to lift objects with the thumb pointing up. Additionally if you manipulate the wrist away from the thumb side of the wrist, you will reproduce the pain. Management may include resting with a splint, ice, and naproxen or ibuprofen. Early office evaluation and consideration for cortisone injection by someone experienced in managing this problem are key. If symptoms persist after several injections and rest, surgery may be considered.

People with TFCC will have persistent pain on the small finger side of the wrist. This pain will be worse with pushing activities like push-ups or with rotation of the wrist. Swelling is not common, but clicking in the outside part of the wrist may be noted. Initial management is rest, with which TFCC will ordinarily resolve. For persistent symptoms, evaluations should include a good history, exam, and X-rays. Persistent cases with greater than 4–6 weeks of symptoms might be treated with a cortisone injection. If symptoms persist beyond that, an MRI should be performed to evaluate for possible surgery by a hand surgeon.

42. What is a ganglion cyst, and what can be done about it?

A ganglion cyst is a collection of fluid beneath the skin from an injured or inflamed joint surface or tendon. Ganglions may be anywhere in the body, but they are more commonly seen around the wrist and in particular on the back of the wrist. Often they are nonpainful, soft swellings that develop without a specific injury. Sometimes they may be painful if the wrist is in certain positions.

People seek evaluation of these because of pain with activities, concern for cancer, or unsightliness. Because the cause is injury, the first treatment should include relative rest from any repetitive activities and the use of ice and or anti-inflammatory medications like ibuprofen or naproxen. Home treatments may also include rupture of these cysts, called the "bible method." Although it is not recommended, this method involves striking the cysts with the binding of a bible to acutely rupture them.

Evaluation in a doctor's office should include examination and X-rays. Doctors may offer drainage with a needle with or without injection of anti-inflammatory steroids. These methods, although effective, run the risk of recurrence of the cyst and might not be satisfactory. Additionally, the injection of corticosteroids under the skin may carry risk of local pigment loss and loss of subcutaneous fat leading to dimpling. The best method to remove the cyst and minimize the chance of recurrence is surgical removal. This surgery is minor, outpatient surgery under local anesthesia performed by an orthopedic surgeon.

Although it is not recommended, this method involves striking the cysts with the binding of a bible to acutely rupture them.

43. What is carpal tunnel syndrome, and how do I treat it?

Carpal tunnel syndrome is the most common overuse nerve condition in the body. Carpal tunnel syndrome involves injury to the median nerve on the palm side of the wrist. This nerve provides sensation to the thumb, index, and middle fingers and strength to the grip of the thumb. This nerve is compressed or pinched from pressure related to fluid accumulation in the carpal tunnel of the wrist, repetitive stretching or pressure on the nerve or acute injury with direct pressure from bleeding. The last is more obvious and associated with wrist fractures or penetrating injuries from a knife or gunshot. The majority of cases are associated with repetitive motions and may include keyboarding, heavy manual work as in construction, or jobs requiring the wrist to be held in the flexed or extended position for a long time. Additionally, certain medical conditions will result in fluid accumulation in the hand such as wrist arthritis, underactive thyroid, pregnancy, and kidney disorders, to name a few.

The most common complaints of people with carpal tunnel are numbness or pain in the thumb, index, or middle finger. Often this is at night or it occurs with their activities at work or recreation. Early on they may be able to alleviate symptoms by merely shaking the hand and changing positions. As symptoms progress they may have more persisting numbness or pain that may even travel up the front of the forearm and develop weakness in the grip, usually noted with attempting to open jars. These symptoms will be further aggravated by wearing any constrictive bands on the wrist as in a tight glove or even a watchband.

Treatments to try at home include changing technique with keyboarding or other activities to avoid prolonged positioning in the extremes of wrist flexion (palm down) or extension (palm back), pressure on the palm side of the wrist on surfaces and avoiding the use of constricting bands on the wrist. Splints to keep the wrist in a neutral position may help maintain proper positioning of the wrist at night and with work or recreational activities. Additionally, one may consider changing the occupational or recreational activity that may be causing problems.

Patients seeking evaluation with a doctor can expect a good hand and wrist examination with neurological testing, X-rays to look for arthritis, and the application of a splint with the initial visit. Subsequent visits may include testing of the nerve function with an Electromyogram (EMG), cortisone injection of the carpal tunnel, and surgery for refractory cases.

Timing of surgery is always a dilemma for patients. With chronic nerve injury we really do not know at what point any nerve damage is irreversible. As symptoms become more chronic, the EMG will help identify at what point nerve damage is occurring and surgery may be indicated. Persistent numbness and weakness with opening jar is a good indication of such damage.

44. What should I do about my thumb injury?

The most common injury to the thumb is the jam injury causing a minor sprain of one of the joints similar to that of the finger as discussed in Question 45. Besides acute fractures, two other common problems of the thumb include the skier's thumb and arthritic problems.

Skier's thumb as it is known today has also been called gamekeeper's thumb in the past. The joint closest to the thumb web space is called the **metacarpal** phalangeal joint. On the web space side of this joint is a very important tendon called the ulnar collateral ligament (UCL). This ligament is injured by falling on the hand with the thumb out or trying to catch a large ball with the thumb out. This ligament gets acutely stretched and may tear or cause a small bone chip if it pulls off the bone. The important part of this injury is recognizing it in order to diagnose and manage it. If you suspect injury to this ligament, have it evaluated in a physician's office by someone familiar with hand problems. X-rays should be taken and usually a splint is applied. If there is a fracture or concern of a complete tear of the ligament, you should see a hand surgeon.

Metacarpal

A bone that connects the wrist to the knuckle of a finger.

Another common complaint either from acute injury or overuse is arthritis. Most commonly this is in the carpal-metacarpal joint of the thumb (**first CMC**). The joint between the base of the thumb and wrist is the first CMC. People who do a lot of manual work, such as carpenters or woodworkers, those who do needlepoint, or those with a history of injury commonly wear this joint out. Often they will have local pain and swelling aggravated by an injury or increased manual

First CMC

The carpal-metacarpal joint of the thumb.

work. Simple home management in the absence of injury would be relative rest for aggravating activities, application of ice, taking naproxen or ibuprofen, and applying a splint. Office evaluation should include examination and X-rays and may include a referral to a hand therapist, application of a splint, and injection of the first CMC with cortisone. For refractory and end-stage cases, a hand surgeon can operate to limit pain and improve pain-free function.

45. What should I do about my jammed finger?

The most common finger injury in sports is the jammed finger. This involves being struck on the end of the finger by a ball, immovable object (wall or tree), or person. When struck on the end with a heavy load, often the proximal interphalangeal (**PIP**) joint will give out. The PIP joint is the one closest to the hand, and the distal interphalangeal joint (**DIP**) is closer to the tip.

PIP

Proximal interphalangeal joint; the finger joint closer to the knuckle.

DIP

Distal interphalangeal joint; the finger joint closest to the finger tip.

When the finger is jammed, the joint surfaces may be injured from crushing, or the joint may dislocate. These dislocations can be obvious with a deformed PIP. The joint might also dislocate or start to dislocate, tearing tissues and self-reducing. When this happens the collateral ligaments (on the sides) or the volar plate (a thickening of the joint capsule on the palm side of the joint) may be torn or they may pull off small chip fractures when injured.

The mainstays of treatment of jammed fingers are ice and relative rest with motion as tolerated and splinting. Persistent deformity, inability to bend the joint, and loss of nerve function indicate need for more urgent evaluation with your doctor or in the emergency room. Minor injuries are indicated by mild swelling and bruising and minimal loss of motion of the joint. These may be treated with ice and ibuprofen for the pain and buddy taping. Buddy taping involves taping the affected finger to the adjacent finger below and above the PIP joint using 0.25-inch cloth or athletic tape. As pain and swelling improve, work on motion by making a fist and squeezing some silly putty or a small ball. When you return to sports, wear the buddy tape for 6 weeks to give support while the tissues are healing.

With jam injuries, if the PIP is not injured the DIP might be. When this occurs, it is called a mallet finger. This often occurs in football, baseball, or basketball. When the finger is struck on the end there is a forceful flexion of the joint causing injury to the tendon that helps keep the joint straight. Besides the acute swelling, you will notice that the end of the finger droops and you will be unable to straighten it out. Although DIP injuries do heal well, they should be evaluated in a doctor's office. X-rays should be taken to look for a fracture and a splint should be applied to keep the DIP straight. When applied, this splint should be worn continuously for 6–8 weeks.

Two other common finger injuries include jersey finger and central slip injuries. Central slip injuries involve injury to the extensor (finger straightening) tendons on top of the PIP joint. These injuries may occur with a dislocation of the PIP toward the palm or a blow or stab injury on top of the PIP. With these injuries, there may be just subtle findings of weakness with attempts to keep the finger straight when a flexing force is applied to the PIP. If not properly cared for, these injuries can result in a permanent deformity called the Boutonnière deformity. With this, the PIP is stuck in flexion and the DIP in extension, rendering the finger minimally functional. Suspicion for such an injury should be evaluated with a provider familiar with hand injuries.

Rather than a jam injury, a jersey finger is a grabbing injury, hence the name. Jersey finger often occurs in tackling sports like rugby or football and usually involves the ring finger because of its importance in grabbing someone's jersey and

Rather than a jam injury, a jersey finger is a grabbing injury, hence the name.

the likelihood that it is the last digit holding onto a jersey in an attempted tackle. The flexor tendon that goes to the end of the finger is torn. With the fingers in the resting position, the affected finger is straight as opposed to mild flexion of the others. Additionally, the player will not be able to bring the finger to the palm as if making a fist. Actual or suspected jersey finger should be evaluated by a provider familiar with hand or sports injuries.

46. What is a subungual hematoma, and how should I treat it?

A subungual hematoma is a blood collection under the nail of a finger or toe. Universally it is caused by trauma. For this reason most people will be able to identify an event that caused it, such as dropping an object on their finger or slamming it in a door. Toe problems can be caused by dropping an object or even by ill-fitting running shoes.

This hematoma is universally painful. It will look like black or dark red discoloration under the nail.

A subungual hematoma will resolve in 4 weeks with most of the pain for the first week if it is left alone. Initial treatment includes the application of ice, as well as acetaminophen, naproxen, or ibuprofen for pain. Draining the hematoma will alleviate this acute pain. If you elect to treat your subungual hematoma at home, all you need is a cigarette lighter and a paper clip. Unfold the clip, making is straight. Cleanse the finger with alcohol or at least soap and water. Use the lighter to heat one end of the paper clip while holding the other end to avoid burning the fingers holding the clip. When the tip is red hot, gently apply it to the center of the nail over the hematoma. The hot clip will burn through the nail with some smoke. It may take one to three applications of the heated paper clip to get fully through the nail. When the hole is through the nail, there will be an instantaneous pain with immediate gush of blood from the hematoma. Express as much blood as will come out and cover with a bandage. Keep the finger clean with soap and water for the next few days, observing for any signs of infection manifested by pus drainage, swelling, pain, and redness of the finger. The nail is destined to fall off in the upcoming weeks. A new nail will start to grow from the nail bed, lifting the old nail. Clip exposed portions as the base of the old nail is elevated and cover with a bandage to avoid catching it. This process will take 4–6 weeks for the new nail to fully grow in and replace the old.

47. What is trigger finger, and what should I do about it?

Trigger fingers are common causes of painful popping of the fingers in people with a history of repetitive gripping with racket sports, golf, manual work, or gardening.

People with trigger finger often sense that their finger is catching or even dislocating when attempting to flex. Another common complaint may include awakening with the finger stuck in the flexed position on the palm and inability to straighten it without a loud pop or significant pain.

Two long tendons help us flex our finger to the palm. The long flexor goes all the way to the end of the finger. If it were not held tightly to the finger, the tendon would bowstring across the palm when we make a fist or flex a finger. There are a series of pulleys that keep the tendon close to the bone of the finger when we make such motions. The first of these pulleys is at the metacarpal phalangeal joint (the MCP, or the knuckle). In the event of repetitive motions and gripping activities, the flexor tendon develops inflammatory nodules. Often this will be near the knuckle joint. If this occurs, bending the finger at the knuckle causes these nodules to become caught on the first pulley, which, in turn, causes painful catching or triggering. Although all the fingers and the thumbs can be affected, this is most common in the ring finger because of its importance in our grip that chronically injures the tendons.

If you develop this triggering, you can try home treatments that include anti-inflammatory medications and application of ice. Additionally, to avoid further tendon injury, you should use a padded glove when doing manual or recreational work that involves gripping.

A doctor might prescribe prescription anti-inflammatory medications, injection, or surgery. Injections of anti-inflammatory steroids are often helpful. These should be limited to two per finger because of the risk of tendon rupture from repeated injections. Surgical procedures, usually performed by an orthopedic surgeon, include releasing the pulley or shaving the inflammatory nodule on the tendon. This is a minor, outpatient procedure.

PART FOUR

Trunk Injuries

I got hit in the ribs, and they really hurt;
what should I do now?

What are side stitches, and what
should I do about them?

What is sciatica, and what should I do about it?

More . . .

48. I got hit in the ribs, and they really hurt; what should I do now?

Blunt injuries to the chest wall may lead to contusion, fractures, costochondral separation or slipped rib, and abdominal injuries. Athletes with these injuries will often complain of severe pain, which is worse with inspiration and direct pressure.

A slipped rib may occur with fracture of the cartilage that holds the rib in place, allowing the rib to intermittently move out of position, with significant pain and popping. Whether subluxed (slipped), contused (bruised), or fractured (broken), despite being quite painful, rib injuries are usually treated conservatively with ice, NSAIDs, and occasionally narcotic pain medications.

Acute rib fracture, however, carries the risk of damage to underlying structures, as the sharp edge of a fractured and displaced rib may puncture or lacerate a lung, the liver, or spleen. Shortness of breath or coughing up blood are both concerning symptoms for damage to the lung. Severe pain associated with chest trauma, particularly abdominal pain, requires examination by a physician to rule out these complications. Without evidence of complications, treatment involves pain control with medications and ice and splinting for comfort. An athlete may return to sports participation with protective padding once his acute injury has been evaluated.

49. I got hit in the abdomen, and it really hurts; what should I do now?

The abdomen is made up of layers of muscle and connective tissue and the abdominal viscera, or organs, that they surround. The abdominal muscles, from exterior to interior, include the rectus abdominus, external and internal obliques, and the transversus abdominus. In addition to governing flexion and assisting with rotation of the trunk, the abdominal muscles support and protect the abdominal viscera, and, particularly the transversus abdominus, which forms a rigid cylinder that supports the spine. The abdominal organs include the liver and gallbladder just below the right costal margin, or lower border of the ribs; the spleen just below the left costal (rib) margin; the stomach and pancreas in the upper central abdomen; the small and large intestine, the bladder, and the kidneys posteriorly. The abdomen is also traversed by the great vessels, or aorta and **inferior** vena cava, which deliver blood to the heart and from the heart, respectively.

Inferior
Below or under.

Muscular soreness after being struck in the abdomen is common. Concern, however, must be given to whether there is damage to underlying organs. Trauma to the upper right or left abdomen may cause damage to the liver and spleen, respectively. This is particularly true if the lower ribs are fractured and displaced, as they may puncture the underlying organs. Trauma to the upper middle abdomen may cause damage to the pancreas, or traumatic pancreatitis. Trauma lower in the abdomen may cause contusion of the bowels, while posterior injury may cause contusion or laceration of the kidneys or ureters.

Seek medical attention if you have pain that radiates to the back, is located in an area different from that in which you were struck, if you have nausea, shortness of breath, sweatiness, or dizziness, if your pain feels deep to the abdominal wall, or is severe. Bruising around the belly button or on the lower back may be a worrisome sign of internal bleeding. Blood in the urine causes concern for damage to the kidneys, ureters, or bladder. These signs usually do not appear for several hours after the injury.

Bruising around the belly button or on the lower back may be a worrisome sign of internal bleeding.

50. What are side stitches, and what should I do about them?

A stitch is typically described as a sharp/stabbing pain that occurs with exercise, just below the ribs, usually on the right side. Stitches occur most commonly with activities involving running. Previously, it was believed that stitches occurred as blood was shunted away from the diaphragm and toward other muscles during exercise. This theory has fallen out of favor, partially because the diaphragm, being a skeletal muscle, should command extra blood supply during exercise in proportion to other muscles. The current belief is that a stitch is caused by stretching of the ligaments that connect the abdominal organs to the diaphragm.

In order to avoid stitches, wait 2–4 hours after a large meal before exercising. Increasing exercise duration and intensity in a progressive fashion may help to minimize symptoms. Developing the abdominal musculature through a solid core strengthening program may also be helpful. In order to alleviate the symptoms from a stitch during exercise, try slowing your pace and leaning forward slightly to decrease the tension on the involved ligaments. Sometimes, using a hand to push upward from below the painful area can give relief by the same mechanism. Dr. Tim Noakes, in his book, *The Lore of Running*, suggests that it may be helpful to alter your breathing patterns to avoid stitches. Two such methods include belly breathing and changing your gait such that you are beginning inhalation and exhalation as your left foot strikes the ground. Many runners begin and end their breathing cycle on the same foot, such that runners may be described as right- or left-footed with regards to breathing. Practicing this altered gait may decrease the frequency that the liver, the heaviest abdominal organ, is displaced downwards while the diaphragm is in its highest position. Belly breathing, or using the abdominal musculature to assist with the effort of breathing, is thought to lessen the movements of the diaphragm relative to the abdominal organs. This may be practiced by lying on your back with an object (book, can, etc.) on your abdomen. Concentrate on using your abdominal muscles to breathe while moving the object up and down as you inhale and exhale.

Abdominal pain that occurs with exercise is not always benign. Abdominal pain sometimes represents angina, or lack of blood flow to the heart, which may precede a heart attack. Pain in the abdomen or back can also be caused by a dissecting aneurysm of the aorta, or intestine that is not getting adequate blood flow. Intestine that does not receive adequate blood flow may die and deteriorate, requiring surgical repair and putting the patient at risk for overwhelming infection. If you have risk factors for heart disease, such as smoking, diabetes, high blood pressure, peripheral vascular disease, obesity, elevated cholesterol, or a family history of heart attack, angina, stroke, or aortic aneurysm, please consult your physician if you have abdominal pain during exercise. Anyone with symptoms that do not seem classical for a stitch, especially symptoms associated with nausea, sweatiness, pallor, and shortness of breath, should also consult his or her physician.

51. What should I do about my back pain?

The bony spine and the muscles and ligaments that support it form the foundation from which all movement of the trunk and extremities originate, and all movements may impart some stress to the back. Because of this fact, back pain is a malady that affects most athletes and nonathletes at some point in their lives. At any one time, approximately 10–25% of the population is suffering from low back pain, with a peak incidence between 45 and 60 years of age. About 80% of all adults seek medical care at some time for low back pain.

The back is an extraordinarily complex anatomical unit. Components include the bony spine, which provides weight-bearing support and protects the spinal cord; disks between the vertebral bodies that provide cushioning; and a complex system of muscles and ligaments that support the bony spine. Because of this anatomical complexity, there are many causes of back pain, including but not limited to muscular strain and deconditioning, disk herniation, arthritis or degenerative changes, spinal canal narrowing or spinal stenosis, fracture, spondylolisthesis or spondylosis, facet pain, and sacroiliac or pelvic joint pain. Back pain that occurs after an injury may be caused by a fracture and should be evaluated by a doctor.

Although back pain is common in the general population, back pain in athletes must be evaluated in a different light. Because of the increased stresses imparted on the back during exercise, athletes are more likely to have back pain secondary to acute muscular strain, ligamentous strain, or fracture. Fractures that must be considered in athletes include compression fractures of the vertebral bodies and fracture of the transverse and spinous processes. Stress imparted by flexion may cause disk herniation, muscular pain, and ligamentous pain. Stresses imparted by hyperextension may cause facet pain, spondylolysis and spondylolisthesis.

Because athletes frequently incur acute injuries that require treatment by a physician, please refer to Question 52. For acute low back pain, bed rest is not helpful, and it often worsens symptoms and delays recovery. An early exercise program to improve mobility often improves symptoms and may decrease time to recovery. Early exercises should focus on stretching and walking. Recommendation for extension or flexion-type stretching often depends on what position causes the most pain (see **Figure 9** on page 179). NSAIDs such as ibuprofen and naproxen may be used for pain relief, as may acetaminophen, heat or ice, and massage. Narcotic pain medications and muscle relaxants may also be employed for pain relief, although neither improves time to recovery. Muscle relaxants have been found to be no more effective than NSAIDs for pain relief. Once the initial severe pain has abated, the recovery and rehabilitation program should focus on a general flexibility and core stability program as discussed in Question 55.

Chronic back pain is commonly associated with obesity, poor posture and muscular deconditioning, and loss of flexibility.

Those with chronic back pain often benefit from weight loss and a regimented rehabilitation program focused on core strengthening and improving back and hamstring flexibility.

52. When should I see a doctor about my back pain?

For muscular low back pain, you should see your physician if your pain is too severe to be controlled by over-the-counter medicines, or if you fail a reasonable (usually 2–6 weeks) course of conservative treatment, as discussed in Question 51. If your pain began as the result of an injury, especially if you have risk factors for osteoporosis, you should see your physician to rule out fracture. Pain that is worse with standing or walking may be suggestive of spinal stenosis. Pain that shoots down your legs, numbness, weakness, or any urinary symptoms may be suggestive of a herniated disk that is compressing a nerve root.

There are a number of types of back pain that are not of musculoskeletal origin. Pain in the lower back associated with blood in the urine may be secondary to kidney stones. This type of pain often makes it uncomfortable to sit still. If you have risk factors for heart or vascular disease, severe back pain may represent an abdominal aneurysm. Infections in the back are rare, but inform your doctor if you have back pain that seems to be related to a fever or associated with a rash. Some cancers spread to bone or cause osteoporosis. If you have back pain associated with weight loss, night sweats, or other symptoms, you should also consult your physician.

53. When should I get X-rays for my back pain?

Back pain that began with an injury may be likely to represent a fracture and should be imaged, especially if there is concomitant osteoporosis or risk thereof. Cancer may metastasize to bone or cause osteoporosis. Chronic back pain with morning stiffness and possibly other swollen, stiff, or painful joints may represent a form of arthritis, ankylosing spondylitis, which is known for the classical X-ray appearance of "bamboo spine." Intermittent pain since the teenage years, possibly at one time worsened by an injury, may represent spondylolisthesis (see Question 18) or the forward displacement of one vertebral body over another. This condition may be caused by spondylolysis, a stress fracture of the pars interarticularis, a portion of the lumbar vertebra (lower back) that articulates with the vertebral body below and stabilizes the two vertebral bodies relative to one another. In its most severe form, this may cause nerve compression and require surgery.

Physicians have identified low back pain red flags for urgent need of X-rays: the very young and old (teenagers and age > 60), personal history of cancer, fever, weight loss, night pains, direct trauma to the back, profound weakness of the legs, or bladder problems. Finally, failure to respond to appropriate therapy in 1 month warrants evaluation.

54. What is sciatica, and what should I do about it?

Sciatica

A term for irritation of the sciatic nerve in the buttocks and leg. Manifested by chronic aching pain the radiates from the buttocks down the leg and is aggravated by sitting or coughing and sneezing. Sciatic pain is the same pain that one with a herniated disc will experience.

Sciatica may be secondary to compression or irritation of a nerve or nerve root, and may occur with disk herniation or other pathologies. The pain of sciatica typically begins in the back or buttock and radiates down the leg, commonly to the back of the thigh and the calf, and sometimes to the foot. Pain that radiates to the knee is less specific to sciatica, but cramping in the leg is common. This pain is frequently described as sharp, or almost electricity-like, and may be associated with numbness, weakness, or tingling in the involved leg. Patients with sciatica prefer to stand as sitting aggravates their symptoms as well valsalva maneuvers (coughing or sneezing) will significantly aggravate or exacerbate their symptoms.

The sciatic nerve is the largest and longest nerve in the human body, and it has the diameter of a finger. Symptoms of sciatica may occur secondary to irritation to the nerve at many levels and has many potential causes. Herniation of a disk may cause compression of the nerve roots as they exit to join the sciatic nerve. Nerve roots may also be compressed by degenerative changes in the bony spine. Especially in individuals whose sciatic nerve travels through the piriformis muscle, muscular pathology or even simple muscle contraction may cause sciatica. Spondylolisthesis and spinal stenosis (see Question 52) may also cause nerve compression and symptoms of sciatica. Disk herniation is most common in the lower spine, and in many with a herniated disk, pain begins while bending or twisting. In the setting of disk herniation, sitting, coughing, or bearing down may make symptoms worse, and standing may provide some relief.

With conservative treatment, sciatica usually resolves within 8–12 weeks. You may treat your pain with ice, acetaminophen, ibuprofen or naproxen. Bed rest is not helpful and may worsen your symptoms. Early rehabilitation programs should be biased toward extension-based exercises and should be followed by a core strengthening program (see Question 55). You should see your physician if you have numbness of your inner thighs, genitals or anus, with severe or increasing weakness, or with any urinary symptoms. Magnetic resonance imaging (MRI) is the preferred way to image the intervertebral disks and soft tissues. Although quite sensitive for disease of these tissues, MRI may identify herniated disks in one quarter to one third of asymptomatic patients, and it should only be obtained as a confirmatory test under certain circumstances. Your physician may decide to obtain an MRI if you have the aforementioned symptoms or if your symptoms do not improve after an appropriate course of conservative therapy.

55. What is all this hype about core stability, and what should I do about it?

The bony spine is a multisegmented column that is unstable by nature and subject to compression and rotation at individual joints unless stabilized. The muscular core includes the muscles that support the spine, the abdominal muscles, the pelvic floor muscles, and the hip muscles. Every motion, not only of the trunk, but also of the limbs, begins in the core. Each motion of an extremity imparts an opposing force to the spine, which in turn is stabilized by the core.

Each motion of an extremity imparts an opposing force to the spine, which in turn is stabilized by the core.

There are shorter muscle groups that provide stability and rigidity of one vertebral body relative to the vertebral body above and below. These shorter muscles also provide a rigid framework that allows the longer spinal muscles that extend the back to function. These longer muscles are opposed by the rectus abdominus but also serve to flex the trunk slowly by slowly relaxing. They play an important role in balancing external loads to minimize the force imparted to the bony spine. Contraction of the innermost abdominal muscle, the transversus abdominus, helps form a rigid cylinder that further supports the spine. Other abdominal muscles work directionally to provide support for specific limb movements. The gluteus maximus, hamstrings, and hip and pelvic muscles provide a base of support for the lumbar spine and upper and lower extremities.

Because the core muscles provide the base from which all movement occurs, improving core strength in athletes is thought to be important not only for enhancing athletic performance, but also for reducing injuries. Several studies have suggested a decreased rate of lower limb injuries with core strengthening programs. Core stability is critically important in patients with back pain. Chronic low back pain may often result from lack of support and stability of vertebrae relative to each other. Loss of rigidity between these levels may cause abnormal mobility in multiple planes.

The goal of a core stability program should be to improve flexibility, strength, and balance. Endurance of muscles to maintain a constant base of stability is more important than pure strength. Basic core flexibility exercises may include hamstring hip flexor, and piriformis muscle stretching as demonstrated in **Figure 10** on page 180. Basic core strengthening exercises may include the pelvic tilt, crunches, bridging, and the quadruped (opposite arm and leg) as demonstrated in **Figure 11** on page 181. Examples of more advanced core stability programs may include pilates or training with a Swiss exercise ball.

Comments from Dr. Susan Burroughs—*Thirty years ago, on the day before my SATs, I twisted to straighten a sheet on my bed and felt a pop on the left side of my back. By the next morning, I had severe left-sided back pain with radiation down my left leg. Rather than attending my SATs I went to the emergency room, where I was given pain medication and muscle relaxants and told to use heat and stay on bed rest until the pain resolved.*

Within 3 or 4 days, my pain was better. I did nothing special to prevent further problems and had no further pain until college. The weekend before final exams in my junior year of college, I took a weekend job that involved heavy lifting. I used my back and not my legs to lift, and by Monday morning, I again had back pain with left-sided radicular symptoms. I was seen in student health and given pain medication and muscle relaxants, but this time was told not to stay on bed rest and was given back exercises. Within 2 days, I was much improved. I continued my exercises faithfully after I recovered and had no further problems through medical school, residency, and two pregnancies.

However, about 5 years ago, I stopped doing my exercises. Within several weeks, I had a recurrence of my symptoms. Having learned my lesson, I resumed my exercises and have done well since. Despite having preached the importance of continued core strengthening to my patients, I didn't really realize how vital preventive exercises were until I lapsed. I am now a believer, and for better or worse can share my personal experience with my patients.

PART FIVE

Lower Extremity Injuries

What should I do about my groin pull?

What is a sports hernia, and what
should be done about it?

What should I do if my hip clicks, pops, or crackles?

More . . .

56. *What should I do about my groin pull?*

Acute pain in the groin is usually caused by muscle pulls or strains, bruises or hematoma, and sprains. These may be best initially treated as follows:

1. *Relative rest*—avoiding quick and painful movements of the hip initially after the injury can be helpful. Specifically, avoid stretching in abducted (legs apart), externally rotated (open frog-legged), and extended (stretching the front of the hip) activities.

2. *Ice versus heat*—the application of ice following the injury can help with pain relief (see Question 10). Later, heat, such as a warm heating pad, can be very useful, especially before starting your rehabilitation exercises or if you feel stiff. Start with ice, and then move to heat. If you reinjure your hip, go back to ice.

3. *Massage*—very gentle massage may help. Do not massage too vigorously, as this may actually prolong your recovery.

4. *Stretching and strengthening*—stretching and strengthening exercises should initially be done gently, and then increased as your groin injury recovers. This speeds healing, alleviates spasm, and helps prevent further injury (see **Figure 12** on page 182).

5. *Medications*—various over-the-counter medications may be helpful (see Question 11).

While the most common cause of groin pain in athletes are muscle or tendon strains, bruises or hematoma, and sprains, there are many injuries and problems that can show up as groin pain, including:

• Hip arthritis, labral tears, and other hip joint problems
• Stress fractures of the pelvis or hip
• Acute hip fractures
• Avascular necrosis of the hip
• Hip dislocations or subluxations

- Various types of hernias (see Question 57)
- Various types of bursitis (see Question 59)
- Testicular or scrotal problems
- Appendicitis and other problems with the intestines
- Urinary tract infections, stones, and other problems with the kidneys
- Nerve problems

Groin strains typically improve within 2 weeks of appropriate care. Diagnosing the cause of hip or groin pain can be difficult. If your groin pain fails to improve with the above treatment, you should seek help from your healthcare professional.

Groin strains typically improve within 2 weeks of appropriate care.

57. What is a sports hernia, and what should be done about it?

A sports hernia, also known as athletic pubalgia, Gilmore's groin, or sportsman's hernia, is caused by a weakness or defect in the wall of lower abdominal muscles that help make up the inguinal canal. This problem may occur in any athlete, but more commonly is seen in cutting sports like soccer, football, rugby, or hockey. The inguinal canal is a soft tissue tunnel in the groin area, through which several structures travel to and from the abdominal cavity. In males, this includes the blood vessels, ducts, and nerves that connect to the scrotum and testicles. In women, the inguinal canal transmits the round ligament, which helps support the uterus, and some nerves as well. The walls of the inguinal canal are made up of contributions from the abdominal muscles (internal and external obliques, and transversalis muscles), the conjoint tendon, and multiple ligaments (inguinal and lacunar ligaments). Holes in these walls can occur. This is the place where many inguinal hernias occur in the groin. Inguinal hernias are true hernias, in which a piece or loop of intestine actually pokes through the soft-tissue walls of the inguinal canal, causing discomfort, pain, or a soft mass in the groin. The hernia may either stay out or go back into the abdomen.

In Gilmore's groin or sportsman's hernia, the intestines do not actually poke through the muscular walls. It is therefore not a true hernia, but there is a weakness or even a minor tear in the walls nonetheless. This causes groin pain, soreness, or stiffness made worse by running, twisting, and squatting activities. Relatively minor movements, coughing, sneezing, or straining may also worsen the symptoms. One theory as to why this happens is that athletes with very strong and tight hip flexor muscles may actually tilt the pelvis down and forward, stretching the abdominal muscles, instead of just flexing the hip. This stretching may weaken the walls of the inguinal canal. After all, Gilmore's groin is more commonly seen in sports where there is a lot of bending or leaning forward and explosive hip flexion, including soccer, hockey, football, rugby, tennis, and track and field. The diagnosis, however, can be very difficult to make, since many problems can present the same way. If there is any question whether you have a sportsman's hernia rather than a regular groin pull, see your healthcare professional.

While some have recommended rehabilitation exercises for strengthening the abdominal, lower back, hip, and pelvic muscles, this condition tends to gradually worsen and progress despite conservative measures. Surgery is often needed to definitively treat this condition if conservative treatment fails to improve symptoms. There are also very specific postoperative rehabilitation exercises. See your healthcare professional if your groin symptoms do not improve.

58. What should I do about my hip pain?

There are many causes of hip pain, depending on where in the hip the pain is. Pain in the posterior (back side) hip or buttock area is commonly caused by bruises (contusions) and hematoma in the soft tissues (muscles, tendons, ligaments) or the bone. This typically responds to rest, ice, gentle stretching, and pain relievers (see PRICEMM in Question 10). It may take 3 weeks or more to see any improvement. Other causes include:

- Back problems, including muscle strains or spasms, ligament sprains, herniated disks, or arthritis (see Question 51)
- Stress or inflammation of the sacroiliac joint between the pelvis and the spine (see Question 51)
- Ischial bursitis
- Coccyx pain
- Avascular necrosis of the hip
- Hip dislocations or subluxations
- Kidney infections, stones, and other problems
- Nerve problems

If you have pain in the back of the hip that does not improve with the above measures, you should be evaluated by a health-care professional.

Lateral (to the side) hip pain is also typically caused by a muscle strain, contusion, or hematoma, and is initially treated the same way posterior hip problems are treated. Other causes include trochanteric bursitis and snapping hip syndrome, which is discussed in Question 59. Another common cause of anterior hip pain is a contusion or hematoma, also called a hip pointer. Hip pointers are treated similar to how hip strains are treated.

Pain in the **anterior** (front) hip is most commonly caused by a hip flexor muscle or tendon strains. This typically responds to rest, ice, gentle stretching, and pain relievers (see PRICEMM in Questions 10 and 11), and may take about 4 weeks or more to see improvement. Occasionally, this injury will be associated with an avulsion fracture, a small piece of bone pulled off of the main bone by a ligament or tendon. These are usually not pulled too far from their attachment and can still be treated conservatively. However, if the fragment is pulled off too much, it may require surgical treatment. There are more concerning injuries that present as anterior hip pain.

Anterior
Toward the front.

Stress fractures can occur about the hip, more commonly in the pelvic bones than the upper thigh bone (femoral neck). General information on stress fractures is discussed in Question 70. Pelvic and femoral neck stress fractures are commonly seen in long-distance runners and military recruits, and they can start out with a deep, vague, achy pain in the anterior hip, become worse during or after activity, and feel better some time after stopping the activity. Pain is typically worse while standing on one leg, unsupported on the injured side. More advanced cases may even cause pain while the athlete walks, causing him or her to walk with a limp. Left untreated, stress fractures can progress to a true, complete fracture with all its complications. Certain types of femoral neck fractures may lead to a condition called avascular necrosis (see next paragraph). If you suspect that you have a stress fracture, see your healthcare professional. He or she will ask you many details about your training habits, equipment, and symptoms. Your healthcare provider will also perform a detailed exam and may order an X-ray or other special tests, such as a bone scan or MRI. Treatment consists of rest—possibly including being non–weight-bearing on crutches—rehabilitation exercises, nutritional measures, and perhaps equipment changes. Some types of femoral neck stress fractures require surgery, since they have a higher chance of progressing to a complete fracture and avascular necrosis (see next paragraph). It can take anywhere from weeks to months for the injury to heal enough for you to return to training. The athlete should gradually resume training, always being ready to back off or even stop if symptoms return.

AVN

Avascular necrosis; bone that loses its blood supply and dies.

Avascular necrosis (**AVN**, also called osteonecrosis) is a condition that interferes with the blood supply to the bone. The bone then becomes starved of nutrients, becomes necrotic and dies, crumbling and becoming very inflamed and painful. Some risk factors for AVN of the hip include femoral neck fractures (either stress or complete fractures), hip dislocations, chronic alcohol use, steroid use (usually chronic, rarely with short-term use), gout, diabetes, sickle cell disease, and other prior injuries to the bones in the hip. Patients with AVN of the hip may experience sudden, incapacitating pain in the anterior hip or groin, which is made worse with bearing weight on the affected side, walking, or simply moving the affected hip. If you suspect you have AVN, see your healthcare professional. He or she will ask you many details about your symptoms, perform a detailed exam, and may order an X-ray or other special tests, such as an MRI. Conservative treatments—such as pain medications, electrical stimulation, and rehabilitation exercises—are rarely successful. Treatment for most cases of AVN is therefore surgical, including procedures to alleviate the pressure inside the bone, bone grafting, and replacing the joint itself. Speak frankly to your healthcare provider or orthopedic surgeon about your treatment options for AVN.

Other causes of anterior hip pain include:

- The same causes of groin pain (see Questions 56 and 57)
- Osteitis pubis (stress or inflammation in the joint between the left and right pubic bones)
- Snapping hip syndrome (see Question 59)
- Arthritis, labral tears, and other hip joint problems (see Question 59)
- Acute hip fractures, dislocations, or subluxations
- Various types of hernias (see Question 57)
- Various types of bursitis (see Question 59)
- Testicular or scrotal problems
- Appendicitis and other problems with the intestines
- Urinary tract infections, stones, and other problems with the kidneys
- Nerve problems

If your injury doesn't respond in a reasonable amount of time, you should see your healthcare provider, who may order an X-ray and recommend other treatment options. Injuries causing mainly groin pain are discussed in Questions 56 and 57.

59. *What should I do if my hip clicks, pops, or crackles?*

There are many things that can cause a popping, snapping, clicking, or cracking sensation in the hip. In general, if these symptoms are not associated with pain, then they may not be significant. The most common cause of these symptoms is snapping hip syndrome.

In the body, there are many places where a muscle or tendon rubs against bony prominences (raised areas of bone). Usually, there is a bursa between the bone and muscle or tendon. A bursa is essentially a flattened balloon or sac, with a drop or two of fluid to make the inside of the bursa slippery. This acts to protect the muscle or tendon from damaging itself from rubbing against the bone. If the muscle or tendon is too tight or inflexible, it can excessively rub against both the bursa and the bone. This is then felt as a snapping or clicking sensation. The whole process can lead to inflammation of the bursa (bursitis) and tendon or muscle, which is then felt as pain. In the hip area, this can occur in the front (anterior) and side (lateral) hip. Lateral snapping hip syndrome is associated with trochanteric bursitis and is also called iliotibial tract (IT) band syndrome in the hip. **Trochanteric bursitis** is a very common hip problem. Anterior snapping hip syndrome is associated with iliopsoas bursitis.

Trochanteric bursitis

Also known as hip bursitis, it is a common problem that causes pain over the outside of the upper thigh.

These two types of snapping hip syndrome are treated with ice, pain medications (see Questions 10 and 11), and specific rehabilitation exercises focused on stretching the tight muscles or tendons (see **Figure 13** on page 184). If you have a significant amount of pain, this may be due to bursitis, which may benefit from a corticosteroid injection from your healthcare provider (see Question 12). See your healthcare professional if you have pain or if your symptoms do not improve after 4 weeks of treatment. Although they are infrequently recommended, there are surgical treatments as well.

Less commonly, snapping hip syndrome can be caused by a labral tear in the hip. This is a tear in the ring-shaped cartilage in the hip joint, and it may require surgical treatment. See your healthcare professional if you suspect you have a labral tear.

60. What should I do about my hamstring/ quadriceps pull (acute or chronic)? How do I treat muscle strains in general?

When an athlete pulls a muscle (muscle strain), muscle fibers are actually torn. How many fibers are torn reflect how severe the strain is, from a mild strain to, rarely, a complete tear of the muscle itself. Risk factors for muscle strains and tears include:

When an athlete pulls a muscle (muscle strain), muscle fibers are actually torn.

- Tight or inflexible muscles (or tendons)
- Improper warm-up
- Age
- Previous injuries to the same muscle
- Muscle fatigue
- Poor conditioning
- Exercising in cold weather
- High-energy running or sprinting
- Jumping activities
- Overuse (doing too much, too soon, too fast)

Muscle strains usually occur when a muscle at risk for injury (see previous list) is subject to a sudden increase in force— usually a force that wants to stretch the muscle—while the muscle itself is trying to contract. This force causes the muscle fibers to tear, resulting in bleeding that can cause bruising and irritation in the muscle. This can result in a significant amount of sharp, tearing, and burning pain, which may later become more deep, achy, and throbbing. There may also be swelling, stiffness, and bruising. The injured muscle will hurt more if the athlete tries to use it. The athlete may find that the muscle is weak, or if the injury is severe, that he or she cannot use the muscle at all. Occasionally, muscle spasm can occur as well. While quadriceps (front of thigh), hamstring (back of thigh), and calf strains are very common, virtually any muscle can be strained, and the treatment is very similar.

The initial treatment is focused on controlling bleeding and swelling in the muscle. This includes rest, ice, compression, and avoidance of using the affected muscle (see PRICEMM in Question 10). This is very important because the more blood that builds up in the muscle, the more severe the injury, and the longer it will take for the athlete to recover. Over-the-counter medications help relieve pain (see Question 11). Do *not* massage the injured muscle. Once the initial bleeding and inflammation reduces (usually after 2–3 days), very gentle stretching exercises may be started, followed by gradually introduced strengthening exercises (see **Figure 14** on page 186 and **Figure 15** on page 188). Once the injury starts to improve (usually after 7 days), you may slowly progress with the stretching and strengthening rehabilitation exercises. While some discomfort is expected with the rehabilitation exercises, there should not be any pain. If any of the exercises actually hurt, either decrease or stop the exercise.

Muscle strains can take weeks to resolve, assuming that the athlete does not reinjure the muscle. Reinjuring a muscle is very easy to do, so you must be very careful not to hurt the muscle again. If you do reinjure the muscle, treatment restarts with the initial treatment. If your muscle strain does not improve with 3 weeks of appropriate treatment, see your healthcare professional.

61. How should I treat a quadriceps contusion?

A quadriceps contusion, caused by an impact (hit) injury to the front of the thigh, is treated in much the same way as a quadriceps strain (see Question 60). If muscle contusions such as these are not treated promptly and appropriately, the resulting damage and bleeding can lead to delayed healing and even other problems in the muscle later on. For example, a history of repeated, significant muscle contusions (especially the quadriceps muscle) can eventually lead to myositis ossificans, a condition in which bone-like calcifications form inside the substance of the muscle, leading to inflammation, pain, swelling, warmth, and a palpable mass. Some of these conditions resolve on their own, but many need surgical treatment to remove the abnormally formed bone.

62. My knees hurt in the front when I run and climb up or down stairs; what should I do?

Pain in the front (anterior) of the knee is the most common type of knee pain seen in all patients under the age of 30 years old who complain of pain not due to traumatic injury.

Common causes of anterior knee pain include tendon problems (either the quadriceps or patellar tendon), bursitis, arthritis, and patellofemoral pain syndrome. In children and young adolescent athletes, Osgood-Schlatter disease and Sinding-Larsen-Johansson syndrome are common causes (see Question 19 for further discussion). If you notice a large, warm, and painful swollen lump or mass, which may feel like it is filled with fluid, you may have bursitis in the knee. This is treated with rest, ice, compression, pain medications, and perhaps a corticosteroid injection (see Questions 10, 11, and 12); see your healthcare provider for this particular problem.

The other common causes of anterior knee pain can be initially self-treated in a very similar fashion. Tendon problems can be tendonitis (tendinosis) or an actual tear. If you are unable to lift your leg and thigh together with your knee straight, you should see your healthcare provider as soon as you can. Otherwise, you can initially treat tendon problems the same way you treat patellofemoral pain syndrome.

Patellofemoral pain syndrome (PFPS) is also known as retropatellar pain, chondromalacia patellae, runner's knee, and moviegoer's knee. While it is the subject of much debate and clinical research, PFPS is thought to be the result of an imbalance in how the quadriceps muscles pull on the knee cap (patella) in order to straighten the knee. Why or how this happens is a complicated issue, and there are many reasons why an athlete may have PFPS. It may also be caused by poor alignment of the lower extremities, or even simply overuse, meaning doing too much, too fast, too soon. This causes the patella to track abnormally, leading to a stress reaction underneath the patella—where it sits in a groove on the thigh bone (femur)—and subsequently, pain. Some of the specific risk factors that contribute to this abnormal patellar tracking include:

- Wide hips (more common in females than males)
- Knock-kneed posture (more common in females than males)
- Frequent deep knee bending activities (such as climbing up steep inclines, deep squats, and deep lunges)
- Overuse (doing too much, too soon, too fast, and not allowing the body to recover adequately from the increased stress)
- Abnormal foot arches—either high-arched (cavus) or flat-arched (planus) feet, as well as early pronators (see Question 76)
- Tight and inflexible hip flexor, hamstring, quadriceps, and calf muscles
- Tight and inflexible iliotibial bands
- Abnormally rotated thigh (femur) or shin (tibia) bones
- Improper running shoes (see Question 76)
- Asymmetrically developed, less conditioned, or weak quadriceps muscles—especially small and weak vastus medialis oblique (VMO), the part of the quadriceps on the **medial** side of the thigh (the side closest to the midline, also called the inside)
- Weak hip external rotator and abductor muscles

Medial

Inside or closer to the midline.

PFPS occurs in the absence of a traumatic injury. The pain is typically worse after walking or running, or when first getting up after sitting down for a long period of time (the so-called theater sign). The pain is also exacerbated by squatting or deep knee bends, and while climbing up and down stairs. There may also be some mild stiffness and a crackling, popping, or grinding sensation when you move your knee. The symptoms of PFPS are typically improved by resting the knee in a relatively straight position. Initial treatment includes PRICEMM (see Question 10), rehabilitation exercises (see **Figure 15** on page 188), and avoidance of deep knee bending activity. This means not sitting with knees bent more than just slightly (not more than 30 degrees), not lunging or squatting, and avoiding stairs. As you recover, you may gradually reintroduce these activities as tolerated. The rehabilitation exercises focus on strengthening and stretching your thigh muscles (hamstrings and quadriceps, especially the VMO), calf muscles, and some of the hip muscles as demonstrated in **Figure 16** on page 191. Some people have also advocated using supplements containing glucosamine-sulfate and chondroitin-sulfate for PFPS (see Question 68). The use of knee braces for PFPS is controversial, and they may or may not work for you.

The use of knee braces for PFPS is controversial, and they may or may not work for you.

In general, you should see some improvement in your PFPS symptoms after 4–6 weeks of treatment. If your pain persists, you should see your healthcare provider. He or she will ask you for details of your training habits, equipment, shoes, and symptoms. Your provider will then perform a detailed exam, looking for anatomic or mechanical abnormalities (see previous list). He or she may then order an X-ray or other tests and develop a treatment plan for you. This may include formalized physical therapy, prescription medications, orthotic devices and shoe recommendations (see Question 76), or a steroid injection (see Questions 12 and 68). Some cases are very difficult to treat, so your healthcare provider may recommend surgical evaluation and treatment. This usually consists of cleaning and smoothing the cartilage between the patella and its groove on the femur with arthroscopy (using cameras and small instruments inserted into tiny incisions). Speak frankly to your physician or orthopedic surgeon about your treatment options, including surgery.

Osgood-Schlatter disease and Sinding-Larsen-Johansson syndrome are caused by inflammation of the bony growth centers at either end of the patellar tendon, right where the tendon attaches to bone. These conditions are well discussed in Question 19.

Comments from Dani Shibla—*My name is Dani Shibla, and I am 14 years old. I am a competitive dancer who dances for 3–4 hours a day. In the fall of 2006 I was diagnosed with PFPS, a very common knee syndrome. This syndrome is where your knee cap moves around too much and the muscles in your legs need strengthening to support your knees. In November, I did physical therapy for 3 weeks and received many exercises to do every day. When I do the exercises the pain isn't as bad as it could be, but when I don't do them the pain increases badly.*

I learned that strengthening the muscles around the knees helps the kneecap stay in place. The pain is usually at its worst when I overuse my knees. The pain comes and goes in different places. It hurts to jump up, land, and climb up stairs, but it doesn't hurt to cross my legs and sit on my feet. I know that overusing my knees could keep me from dancing for the rest of my life, but I still have to learn to limit the overuse of my knees, so I can continue dancing. Sometimes I ask myself if I'm doing too much, but I know if I do the exercises and do what the doctor tells me too, then I will be able to continue dancing.

63. How should I treat my medial collateral ligament sprain?

The medial collateral ligament (MCL) is one of the major ligaments that stabilize the entire knee joint, and it is located on the medial part of the knee (the side of knee closest to the midline, often called the inside of the knee). The MCL is often injured (sprained) by a direct blow to the lateral side (the side of the knee away from the midline, often called the outside of the knee) with the foot planted. This causes the MCL to stretch, partially tearing its fibers, or even completely tearing it. The same stress to the MCL can result from a twisting injury, or even without the foot planted. Traumatic MCL sprains are very common in football, soccer, and lacrosse. There is a chronic MCL strain seen in swimmers called breaststroker's knee (see Question 89).

Symptoms include pain localized to the medial side of the knee, swelling, and even a wobbly or unstable feeling in the knee. The pain is usually worse with the knee fully straight or bent, and with any twisting activity. There may be other injuries to the knee, with other symptoms as well.

Injuries to the MCL are graded as grade 1, 2, or 3, with grade 3 being a complete tear that may require surgery to fix. In general, the athlete with MCL sprains should seek the attention of an athletic trainer, physician, or other healthcare professional for evaluation, as other, more serious injuries may be present. The healthcare provider will perform an examination, and perhaps order an X-ray or other tests. Treatment typically involves PRICEMM (see Question 10), and perhaps a hinged knee brace to prevent further injury to the MCL. Some providers may recommend general knee rehabilitation exercises or physical therapy as well. Mild sprains improve in 4 weeks, and more severe grade 2 sprains may take 2–3 months to heal. Grade 3 injuries may or may not heal with bracing; some require surgical treatment.

64. What should I do about my anterior cruciate ligament sprain?

The anterior cruciate ligament (ACL) is one of the major, stabilizing ligaments of the knee that helps hold the knee together, especially while in motion. The ACL can be injured when a direct blow to the lateral (outside of the knee), medial (inside of the knee), or anterior (front of the knee) aspect of the knee with the foot planted forces the knee to twist, buckle, or straighten. This causes the ACL to stretch, partially tearing its fibers, or even completely severing it. ACL sprains are very common in football, soccer, lacrosse, and skiing. It usually takes a lot of force to tear an ACL.

Patients may describe hearing or feeling a pop or snap in the knee. Other symptoms include pain over a larger area of the knee, massive amounts of swelling, and even a wobbly or unstable feeling in the knee. Patients will frequently have trouble just putting weight on the leg of the injured side. There may be other injuries to the knee, with other symptoms as well. Athletes with old, chronic, unfixed ACL sprains may have occasional pain and swelling, as well as a buckling or giving way sensation with twisting or turning movements.

Injuries to the ACL are graded as grade 1, 2, or 3. While there are different severity levels to ACL sprains, these injuries typically do not heal on their own and are considered to be severe injuries. If you injure your ACL, you should see a healthcare professional for evaluation. The healthcare provider will perform an examination and perhaps order an X-ray or other tests. An MRI may be recommended to look more closely at the ligaments and cartilages of the knee. Initial treatment typically involves PRICEMM (see Question 10) and perhaps a knee immobilizer or hinged knee brace to prevent further injury, while you and your physician work to decrease the swelling. Some providers recommend physical therapy to help control this swelling. This is very important, because if you need surgery, most surgeons prefer to operate when the swelling is well controlled to prevent wound problems after the surgery.

While bracing and conservative treatments can be used, surgery may be necessary for this condition. Since the ACL helps with stabilizing the knee in a very specific direction, some athletes do reasonably well without surgery, if their knees are only used for certain activities (like running in a straight line) and are stable in the other directions. These patients are usually treated with rehabilitation exercises, physical therapy, and a specific type of knee brace. Pivoting or turning activities, such as those required in basketball, football, or soccer, generally require the ACL to stabilize the knee in order to do the activity, so athletes with ACL injuries who participate in these activities may need surgery. Every patient is unique, and more mild ACL sprains may not require surgery, even in this group. It is ideal to speak frankly with your healthcare provider about risks and benefits of choosing conservative versus surgical treatments. If you elect to not have surgery, you will likely be able to slowly return to sports between 6 and 12 weeks after the injury.

Since a severely injured ACL cannot heal on its own, surgery is focused on reconstructing (replacing) the ACL. There are many techniques and approaches to accomplishing this, including using tendons from other areas in your own body, or a donated tendon or ligament from a cadaver. The surgeon may use arthroscopy (using cameras and small instruments inserted into tiny incisions) or a larger incision to reconstruct the ACL. If you decide on surgery, talk frankly about your options with your orthopedic surgeon. After surgery, postoperative physical therapy is very important in how soon you can return to sports, usually between 6 months and a year after surgery.

Besides having possible problems using the knee after an ACL injury, another concern is that patients who have injured their ACL are at higher risk of developing early arthritis (osteoarthritis). For more information on arthritis, see Question 68. There is much debate as to why this happens. Some think that the resulting motion between the bones of the knee after losing the stabilizing force of the ACL causes arthritis.

Besides having possible problems using the knee after an ACL injury, another concern is that patients who have injured their ACL are at higher risk of developing early arthritis (osteoarthritis).

Others believe that the cartilage on the bones themselves is directly injured from the same injury that caused the ACL tear, and that this injury develops into arthritis (posttraumatic arthritis). Either way, it is important to realize this increased risk of arthritis, so if you have a history of an ACL tear, you can expect long-term knee problems down the road.

The best way to prevent ACL injuries is currently a topic of much debate and research. There are several different approaches and programs used to prevent ACL injuries. As we learn more about what things we can change to decrease the chances an athlete will have an ACL injury, new devices, exercises, and programs will be developed. Here are two of the more popular programs at this time:

- The PEP program. Information is available at http://aclprevent.com/
- The Sportsmetrics program. Information is available at http://www.sportsmetrics.net/

65. When should I see my doctor for my knee injury?

While there are many types of athletic knee problems, most will improve with conservative treatment alone. However, anyone with a knee injury should seek medical attention if:

- There is immediate swelling after the injury
- The injured person cannot put any weight on the affected knee
- There is a buckling or giving way sensation in the knee
- The knee gets locked in a certain position
- There is any numbness, tingling, or persistent weakness in the leg below the knee
- There is any suspicion of a broken bone or dislocation
- There is excruciating pain that the injured person cannot tolerate
- The injury fails to improve with conservative measures

66. *What should I do if my knee clicks, pops, or crackles?*

In general, if the knee has **crepitus** (clicking, popping, or crackling sensations with movement), and there is no pain, there is no significant injury that needs to be treated. If there is pain, the knee should be examined by a healthcare professional familiar with knee problems. A number of problems can cause knee crepitus with pain, including fractures (broken bones), loose pieces of bone or cartilage in the joint, arthritis, and snapping knee syndrome. Some of these cannot be treated conservatively and require surgery.

Crepitus

Grinding that can be felt or heard in a tendon or joint.

67. *What is a cartilage tear and what should be done about it?*

In the knee, sandwiched between the ends of the femur (thigh bone) and tibia (shin bone) are two round, C-shaped pieces of cartilage. These are the menisci (singular, **meniscus**) of the knee, one lateral (outside of the knee) and one medial (inside of the knee). The menisci serve several functions, including shock absorption, stability of the knee, and even distribution of weight across a joint. The menisci can be injured by any action that forces the knee to twist, buckle, bend, or straighten. This can cause the bones of the knee to compress down on and shear the menisci, leading to meniscal tears. Unlike ACL tears, however, it takes less force to tear a meniscus. These injuries are most common in football, soccer, lacrosse, rugby, basketball, and wrestling. Additionally, because menisci help with weight bearing and shock absorption in the knee, they can also gradually wear out in certain places, leading to more chronic, degenerative (wear-and-tear) tears.

Meniscus

The two crescent cartilage cushions in the knee.

Patients with meniscal tears can have a mild to moderate amount of swelling in the knee, as well as pain localized to the side of the knee that has the injured meniscus (lateral or medial). This pain is worse with bending and straightening the knee. Larger tears can also cause a catching, clicking, or popping sensation in the knee. The knee may even become locked in a certain position, being unable to straighten beyond that point.

There are many different types of meniscal tears. The most useful way of thinking about these injuries is to split them up into three groups. Tears along the innermost part of the C-shaped meniscus are central (or white-white) meniscal tears. Tears along the outermost part are called peripheral (or red-red) meniscal tears. Then there are tears in between these two areas, sometimes called red-white meniscal tears. This is important because some meniscal tears, especially peripheral tears, can heal on their own. These injuries do not require surgery. Other meniscal tears, however, require surgical treatment. Unfortunately, there is often no way of knowing which of the three types of injury an athlete has, short of surgery. Because of this, meniscal injuries are initially treated with relative rest and rehabilitation exercises to see if it heals on its own. Athletes with meniscal tears should see a healthcare professional for evaluation. The healthcare provider will perform an examination and perhaps order an X-ray or other tests. An MRI may be recommended to look more closely at the menisci, as well as the ligaments and cartilages of the knee. Initial treatment typically involves PRICEMM (see Question 10) and perhaps a knee brace for comfort. Some providers may recommend physical therapy as well. Either way, you should follow up closely with your healthcare professional until you are well on your way to recovery, which can take between 6 and 12 weeks.

While conservative treatment is often successful in treating meniscal injuries, some meniscal tears do not heal on their own, and surgery may be necessary for this condition. Surgery is focused on repairing those meniscal tears that may still be able to heal or on removing the torn pieces of those that cannot heal (central meniscal tears). The surgeon may use arthroscopy (using cameras and small instruments inserted into tiny incisions) or a larger incision to repair the meniscus. Trimming off torn pieces of the meniscus is usually done through arthroscopy only. Before you decide on surgery, talk frankly about your options with your orthopedic surgeon. After surgery, postoperative physical therapy is very important in determining how soon you can return to sports.

68. What should I do about knee arthritis?

Arthritis is generically any inflammation within a joint. There are many types of arthritis, but the most common one by far is osteoarthritis (OA). This is what most people mean by the term *arthritis*. When two bones meet to make a joint, the surfaces of the bone are usually covered by a special type of slippery cartilage called articular cartilage. This allows the bones to glide past each other with very little friction and no pain. This cartilage also serves as a mild shock absorber. The inside of the joint is also lined with a tissue called synovium, which makes a small amount of fluid that lubricates the joint. OA is a degenerative (or wear-and-tear) condition in which the articular cartilage is worn thin. This can cause the stress across the joint to increase and the cartilage to further thin and crack. The bone underneath the cartilage also feels more stress and starts forming bone spurs. In addition, the synovium can get inflamed and irritated, causing it to make more fluid than it normally does, which can then lead to swelling in the knee. Sometimes, small pieces of cartilage or bone can break off, float into the joint, and cause more inflammation and pain, or even block how the joint moves. OA is often a gradual, slow process. Occasionally, it can flare up with more inflammation, but overall, the condition worsens slowly. When it becomes more severe, it is also called degenerative joint disease (DJD). In some cases, OA may occur due to a preexisting injury to the articular cartilage and is called posttraumatic arthritis. In these injuries, the onset of OA is delayed and may not become evident for many years from the injury, but it occurs earlier than it would had the joint not been injured.

Patients with OA have a deep, dull, achy type of pain in the affected joints. Where the pain in OA comes from is a controversial issue. It may come from the bone under the articular cartilage, the synovium, or even the stretching of the joint from too much synovial fluid. OA pain is more likely a combination of many things. Occasionally, arthritic joints with long-standing OA can flare up and become more inflamed, leading to a more sharp, burning, and throbbing pain. In additional to pain, arthritic joints may also be stiff. This can range from mild to severe, and is usually worst upon awakening in the morning and loosens up within 30–60 minutes of walking about. Symptoms of OA are also typically worse after having used the affected joints all day. Again, there can be a significant amount of swelling in the affected joints as well. In advanced DJD, the articular cartilage can be so worn that the joint is essentially bone-on-bone, and the symptoms can be very severe and debilitating. In fact, some patients can scarcely use the affected joints at all.

In general, you will benefit from evaluation and treatment plans from a healthcare professional. The healthcare provider will perform an examination and perhaps order an X-ray or other tests. He or she will then help you formulate a treatment plan. The following treatment options are specific for the knee, but may be applicable to other joints with OA.

If there is significant swelling within the joint (called an effusion), the provider may recommend taking the fluid out with a needle.

If there is significant swelling within the joint (called an effusion), the provider may recommend taking the fluid out with a needle. This may make your knee feel better and may help in the diagnosis. The physician may want to perform other tests on the removed fluid. Initial treatment includes PRICEMM (see Question 10), especially when the joint is acutely flared up. Overall however, relative rest for OA should be for no more than 24 hours. For the more chronic, achy pain of OA, moist heat usually helps. However, ice may be more helpful than heat for acutely inflamed OA flare-ups. The best approach is to try using both and see which one works best for you.

Acetaminophen at higher doses (up to a total of 4000 mg a day) as well as various over-the-counter and prescription NSAIDs are typically very effective in controlling the pain of OA (see Question 11). Your healthcare provider may also discuss using topical pain medications as well.

Specific rehabilitation exercises focused on the flexibility, strength, and coordination of the muscles that support the knee may also be helpful. Refer to the general knee rehab exercises in **Figure 15** on page 188. Fitness is important for maintaining the health of the existing joint, but individuals should consider cross-training with lower impact exercises like treadmill walking, using an elliptical trainer, biking, swimming, or using a stair machine. Some healthcare providers may recommend working with a physical therapist as well.

Since OA is often a result of increased stress across the affected joint, measures to decrease that stress may provide some relief and allow any flare-ups to resolve. If you are overweight, your healthcare provider may recommend lifestyle changes, such as diet and exercise, to decrease your body weight as a means of relieving the stress on an arthritic joint. Medical devices can also help unload arthritic joints. These include shock-absorbing shoes, orthotic inserts, a cane or walker, splints, and braces. Talk with your healthcare provider for the approach that is best for you.

If your OA symptoms are not improved with the measures just described, your physician may recommend an injection into the affected joint. There are different types of medications that can be injected into the arthritic joint, including local anesthetics (to temporarily numb the pain), corticosteroids (to decrease the inflammation) (see Question 12), and a group of substances called viscosupplements. Viscosupplements are similar to the building block molecules that make up articular cartilage. However, experts are not sure how these substances work. Some patients find good relief of their symptoms with viscosupplementation, while others find little or no relief. Speak frankly with your physician about joint injections, their potential risks and benefits, and which medications may work best for you.

In recent years, there has been much interest in and discussion over the use of glucosamine and chondroitin oral supplements (glucosamine-chondroitin). With several research studies showing mixed results, how effective glucosamine and chondroitin are is very controversial. The two compounds are also building blocks for articular cartilage, but experts do not know how the supplement works to relieve OA pain. Some patients respond well to glucosamine-chondroitin, while others do not. Among the potential side effects, the most common is some upset stomach, and anyone with shellfish allergy should not take this supplement at all. In the United States, glucosamine-chondroitin is currently available as an over-the-counter supplement. There are prescription versions, but these are only available in other countries. Glucosamine-hydrocholoride and chondroitin-sulfate preparations may be more effective than glucosamine-sulfate and chondroitin-HCL preparations. Take a total of 1500 mg of glucosamine and 1200 mg of chondroitin a day. It may take a while for you to realize a full effect of these supplements, so give them 3–6 months of daily use before deciding whether glucosamine-chondroitin preparations work for you.

Finally, if your DJD is advanced and your symptoms have become debilitating, your healthcare provider may recommend surgical treatments. These range from cleaning and smoothing the inside of the arthritic joint with arthroscopy (using cameras and small instruments inserted into tiny incisions) to more invasive, prosthetic joint replacement. Whether or not you need surgery is up to how you feel and how debilitating your symptoms are. Every procedure has its own risks and benefits. Talk frankly with your healthcare provider and orthopedic surgeon about whether you should have a surgical procedure for your OA.

69. *What should I do about shin splints?*

Shin pain is very common in running and jumping sports. They are especially common in athletes who do too much, too soon, too often, and too fast (overuse). The most common cause of shin pain in running is shin splints, also called medial tibial stress syndrome (MTSS). This is thought to occur because of increased stress on the muscles in the back of the leg where they attach to the back of the shin bone (tibia). These muscles include the ones that help you push off when you run or jump. When they are overworked as in an overuse situation, there can be inflammation in the muscles, tendons, and even the bony parts involved in pushing the ankle, foot, and toes down (like pushing on a gas pedal of a car). This, in turn, can cause pain up and down the shin.

Patients with very early or mild cases of MTSS will develop shin or leg pain after activity that goes away with rest. This pain may be made worse when the athlete tries to push off or jump off of the affected leg. Slightly more significant cases of MTSS will involve development of symptoms at the start of activity that decrease during activity and return at the end of activity. More significant cases will include development of symptoms early in the activity and persistence of symptoms throughout the activity. In the most severe cases of MTSS, symptoms can limit the quality and amount of training and even prevent the athlete from training at all. In addition, certain foot and ankle shapes and mechanics, such as flat feet or tight calf muscles, can make it easier for the athlete to get MTSS. Poorly fitted shoes or shoes that are not right for the athlete's foot type can also put him or her at risk for MTSS.

The best first step to treat MTSS is to back off the training, and perhaps even rest without training for a week before very gradually returning to running or jumping. Choosing the right shoes can be important. Specialty running shoe stores are a good place to start; expect the staff to spend anywhere from 15 to 45 minutes helping you find the right shoe for your activities. Orthotic inserts may also be helpful, and there are many over-the-counter inserts that work well. Ask your foot care professional about these as well. Stretching the different calf muscles is also often helpful in treating and preventing MTSS (see **Figure 17** on page 194). The use of oral medications and PRICEMM (see Question 10) may or may not help. Once your symptoms improve, consider cross-training, working on balance and coordination. This may help prevent your MTSS from coming back. An experienced physical therapist, athletic trainer, or personal trainer can help you learn some of these exercises.

If you do not improve with the aforementioned measures, seek the attention of a healthcare professional. He or she will perform a detailed examination, ask about your training habits, equipment, and surfaces, and may order X-rays or other tests. Your healthcare provider will then detail a treatment plan right for you and follow you closely. How soon you will improve will truly depend on your specific situation, but most athletes see an improvement with 3–4 weeks of appropriate care.

There are other conditions that may present in a way very similar to MTSS, including stress fractures in the bones of the leg and compartment syndrome (see Questions 70 and 71). If you think you have a stress fracture, consult your healthcare provider for further evaluation.

70. What exactly is a stress fracture? What should I do about it? What are high-risk stress fractures in runners?

A stress fracture is a series of tiny cracks (microfractures) in the surface of a bone, caused by repetitive, rhythmic, overloading activities, such as running, hiking, marching, dancing, or jumping. This is different from a complete fracture, which is a larger, complete crack, break, or shattering of the bone, through and through. The danger of having an untreated stress fracture is that it can progress to a complete fracture. There are two theories on why stress fractures occur:

Fatigue theory: When muscles tire or fatigue, they can no longer assist in supporting the skeleton as efficiently as they can when they are rested. During repetitive activities that exhaust the muscles, an increased load is placed upon the bones. When the bone's ability to resist these forces is exceeded, tiny cracks develop on its surface.

Overload theory: Muscle contractions exert a pulling force on the bones to which they attach. For example, the contraction of the calf muscles causes the tibia (shin bone) to bend forward like a drawn bow. The repetitive, back-and-forward bowing of the tibia can cause cracks to appear in the front of the tibia.

Most stress fractures are probably a result of a combination of both these problems. Bone has the ability to gradually adapt to the increased stresses of exercise. When the stressors of exercise exceed the bone's ability to compensate and adapt, stress fractures can occur. This is why overuse situations (doing too much, too soon, too fast) often result in stress fractures. Thinner bones are at greatest risk of developing stress fractures. Insufficient bone calcification, as may occur in women with irregular menstrual cycles and certain abnormal eating practices, increases the risk of stress fractures.

Thinner bones are at greatest risk of developing stress fractures.

Other risk factors for stress fractures include several of the same risk factors for shin splints (see Question 69)—change in training shoes, poorly fitted shoes, and change to a different or harder training surface. Athletes doing more high-impact activities are also at higher risk. Those with certain leg, ankle, and foot shapes and mechanics—such as flat feet, high-arched feet, and uneven limb lengths—are at risk for stress fractures as well.

The most common places for a stress fracture include the shin bone (tibia), fibula (outer leg bone), and several bones in the foot and ankle. Symptoms of a stress fracture include dull or sharp pain, usually focused in on specific spots. In mild cases, the pain occurs after activity. More moderate cases will have pain during activity, and the more severe cases will have pain that prevents the athlete from training. There may also be some swelling.

If you suspect that you have a stress fracture, see your healthcare professional. He or she will perform a detailed examination, ask about your training habits, equipment, and surfaces, and may order X-rays, a bone scan, or other tests. Your healthcare provider will then detail a treatment plan for you and follow you closely. Treatment of stress fracture usually includes PRICEMM (see Question 10), stopping pain-producing activities, perhaps bracing, or possibly even crutches. Rehabilitation exercises are important, and your healthcare provider may also recommend physical therapy. Nutrition, calcium, and vitamin C and D supplements may also be helpful. However, rest is probably the most important thing you can do for this condition. How soon you will improve will truly depend on your specific situation, but most athletes see an improvement with 4–6 weeks of appropriate care.

There are other conditions that may present in a way very similar to stress fractures, including shin splints and compartment syndrome (see Questions 69 and 70). If there is any doubt as to your diagnosis, consult your healthcare provider for further evaluation.

71. What should I do about my calf pain?

There are many causes to calf pain in athletes, the most common of which is a muscle strain in the calf. Athletes with a calf strain often report a history of a sudden, sharp pain in the calf that usually interferes with the sporting activity. The athlete may also feel as if he or she was hit in the calf or feel a pop in the calf. Intense pain and swelling develop within 24 hours after the injury, and pain and stiffness are made worse with walking. To keep recovery time to a minimum, it is very important to initiate treatment as soon as possible. See Question 60 for some general treatment pointers for muscle strains. The rehabilitation exercises are also shown in **Figure 18** on page 196. A brace or heel lift may also be helpful in decreasing the stress to the injured muscle. These are available at many sports equipment stores. In general, recovery from a calf strain may take between 3 and 12 weeks. If you see little or no improvement in your symptoms after 3 weeks of appropriate self-treatment, see your healthcare provider. Athletes with tight hamstring and calf muscles are at higher risk of developing calf strains, so maintaining your flexibility is important.

Some other causes of calf pain in athletes include:

- Exertional compartment syndrome (ECS): This is a pressure increase in various parts of the leg, usually occurring during or after exercise. Symptoms include deep, achy, squeezing, or sharp pain made better after a longer period of rest (30 minutes to several hours). Muscles may feel weak and even stop working altogether. The leg or foot may have numbness or tingling as well, and the leg may feel very tight, tense, or hard. If you suspect that you have ECS, see your healthcare provider. He or she will perform an examination and may order special tests. There are conservative and surgical treatments, but most athletes benefit most from surgery.
- Stress fractures: See Question 70.
- Blood clots or compressed blood vessels in the leg: These are very dangerous conditions that require evaluation and treatment from a physician sooner rather than later. Symptoms include cramping, achy leg pain with exercise, but no symptoms at rest. These symptoms can resemble those of ECS, except that ECS symptoms tend to persist for about 30 minutes after stopping the

activity. Exercise-related compression of the blood vessels tends to have pain that resolves within a few minutes of stopping the activity. Your healthcare provider will perform a detailed examination and order special tests. Treatment depends on the specific cause, but it may include blood-thinning medications, medications used to open up the blood vessels, or even surgery.

72. What should I do about my sprained ankle?

Sprained ankles are very common in sports participation and exercise activities, especially basketball, volleyball, tennis, football, soccer, wrestling, martial arts, and other jumping sports. There are mainly three groups of ligaments in the ankle, including the medial (the side closest to the midline), lateral (the side farthest from the midline), and a third group made up of all the ligaments in between. In addition, there are tendons on either side of the ankle that can also be injured.

There are several ways to sprain your ankle, usually involving landing from a jump, sudden cutting or pivoting movements, or stepping or landing on an uneven surface. These usually cause the ankle to twist in either direction, flex either up or down with a lot of force, or roll over towards either side of the ankle. This in turn causes the ligaments to stretch and either partially or completely tear. Symptoms of an ankle sprain include pain, bruising, and swelling with some resulting stiffness. These are made worse with walking and running activities. In general, athletes with mild to moderate ankle sprains are still able to bear weight on the affected leg or walk, albeit with a limp. However, there may be more significant injuries, including a broken bone (fracture) or if the ligaments between the medial and lateral ligaments are injured. These may present with the athlete being unable to bear weight or walk without crutches.

Initial treatment for most ankle sprains includes PRICEMM and pain medications (see Questions 10 and 11). There are several ankle braces commercially available to help protect the ankle as it heals. Once the pain and swelling improve (usually after 1–2 weeks), you should start specific rehabilitation exercises to help speed recovery and return to activity, as well as to prevent further injuries. Overall, the rehabilitation of ankle sprains is divided into five phases (see **Figure 19** on page 198). If your ankle fails to improve after 2–3 weeks of the aforementioned treatment, you should see your healthcare professional (see Question 73). Sometimes, an ankle sprain will also result in an injury of either the foot or the area between the foot and the ankle. These are usually more severe injuries and should be evaluated by a healthcare provider as well. Also, if you find that you cannot walk without crutches, or put any weight on the affected ankle or foot, you should see your healthcare provider.

Comments from Caitlyn Jones—*My perspective as an athlete going through physical therapy is that it helped motivate me for a quick recovery. First, I met with the physical therapist so she could evaluate my ankle injury and prescribe a treatment plan. She tested my ankle's range of motion, how strong it was, and how flexible it was. During the first week, the therapist used a combination of heat and active range of motion exercises. In the second week, I worked on my proprioception by standing on a balance board for about a minute; then repeating it three times. I also ran on the treadmill for 10 minutes just as a warm-up prior to doing more strengthening exercises. I was able to improve my ankle's flexibility by outlining the alphabet against the resistance of an elastic rubber band. At home, I worked on my strength and coordination by balancing my weight, standing on one foot. This was very difficult initially, but long term, has helped to stabilize my ankle. The therapist said that if I continued to do these exercises on a daily basis, it would make my ankle become stronger and I would be able to continue my power tumbling. For me physical* *therapy has helped tremendously and that's why I can still keep up with my athletics today.*

73. When should I see a doctor about my ankle pain?

Since some ankle injuries are more severe or complicated to treat than others, it is important to know when you should seek consultation with a healthcare professional familiar with ankle injuries. You should seek professional help if you notice:

- You are unable to put weight on the injured ankle
- Your ankle injury also causes pain elsewhere, such as the upper leg or foot
- Your ankle feels wobbly or loose
- You have numbness, tingling, loss of color, or weakness further down the ankle or foot, or if these areas are cool to the touch in the absence of using ice
- Your pain is very severe and unbearable
- You have areas of the leg, ankle, or foot that are exceedingly tight, tense, and hard, and they remain so despite rest and PRICEMM (see Question 10)
- You are older than 50 years old
- Your injury does not improve within a reasonable amount of time using standard, appropriate self-treatment (see Question 72)

A specific type of ankle brace may be recommended, and you might even require crutches to adequately rest your injury.

Once you see your healthcare professional, he or she will perform a detailed examination, ask about your training habits, equipment, surfaces, and how you injured your ankle. He or she may order X-rays, an MRI, or other tests as well. Your healthcare provider will then detail a treatment plan that is right for you and follow you closely. A specific type of ankle brace may be recommended, and you might even require crutches to adequately rest your injury. Rehabilitation exercises are important, and your healthcare provider may also recommend physical therapy. Some types of ankle sprains are considered unstable and may require surgical treatment. Speak frankly to your healthcare provider about treatment options.

74. What should I do about my Achilles tendon injury?

The **Achilles tendon** is the tendon that connects the larger muscles of the calf to the back of the heel bone (calcaneus). Although it is a thick and typically strong tendon, it is subjected to a lot of force both in everyday activities and during sports and exercise, putting the Achilles tendon at risk for inflammation or tears. There is also an area within the tendon that is more vulnerable to injury as well.

Achilles tendon

The large tendon in the back of the heel.

Achilles tendon injuries can be divided into two types: chronic, overuse injuries, and acute injuries. Overuse (doing too much, too soon, too fast) can cause the Achilles tendon to slowly break down; this is called Achilles tendinosis. Symptoms include pain, swelling, and stiffness focused to a specific area (usually about an inch from where it attaches to the calcaneus). If overuse has been occurring for some time, the tendon itself may be thickened and hard. Other risk factors include a recent change in training shoes or training habits, tight hamstring and calf muscles, and certain foot shapes and mechanics (such as a flat foot). Initial treatment may include avoidance of offending activities and relative rest. Avoid running up hills. Orthotic inserts may be helpful if you have flat feet, and a heel lift will often relieve some of the pain. There are specific rehabilitation exercises that may be helpful as well (see **Figure 18** on page 196). Many patients improve after 4–6 weeks of this treatment. If you find no improvement, see your healthcare provider. Severe cases may require a cast or brace, and you may need crutches to adequately rest the tendon if your injury is bad enough. Physical therapy may also be needed. If your symptoms persist, your physician may recommend other treatments. In general, surgical treatment is an option if symptoms persist for 3 months despite good rehabilitation exercises, including physical therapy.

More acute Achilles tendon injuries include tendonitis, partial tears, and complete tears (complete ruptures) of the Achilles tendon. These injuries may occur after a sudden stress is applied to the ankle or foot, forcing it to bend upwards, towards the head. This results in a stretching or even a tear of the Achilles tendon, with bleeding and inflammation. This is very common in sports such as basketball, baseball, tennis, hiking, and soccer. Athletes aged 40–60 years old are at greatest risk. Other risk factors include a history of Achilles tendinosis in the past, the use of certain antibiotics, and a history of prior Achilles tendon tears. You may notice a pop or a feeling as if someone kicked the back of your heel during the sporting activity. This is then followed by focused pain, swelling, stiffness, and perhaps bruising along the Achilles tendon or the back of the heel. This may make it difficult to walk or even to simply put weight on the affected foot and ankle. The initial treatment includes PRICEMM and pain medications (see Questions 10 and 11). A cast, brace, or splint that prevents you from stretching the injured Achilles tendon may help. Heel lifts may be helpful in more mild cases. You may even need crutches to adequately rest the injured tendon. When you begin to feel better, you should start rehabilitation exercises that work on stretching and strengthening the Achilles tendon and calf muscles. If you do not see improvement after 2–3 weeks of self-treatment, see your healthcare provider. He or she will then perform a detailed examination, order an X-ray or other special tests, and put together a good treatment plan for you. Complete tears of the Achilles tendon generally need surgery; speak openly and frankly with your orthopedic surgeon about your options.

75. What should I do about my heel pain?

There are several different causes of heel pain in athletes, the most common of which are heel pad contusions, plantar fasciitis, and heel fat pad atrophy. These conditions present with pain on the bottom of the heel. Pain in the back of the heel is discussed elsewhere in this book (see Question 74).

Heel pad contusions are basically bruises that develop from injury to the fat pad underneath the heel. These injuries are common in martial arts and gymnastics. Hard landings, stomping, or hard-stepping onto a hard surface—such as a hardwood floor or balance beam—can break small blood vessels in the heel fat pad. The resulting bleeding causes pain on the bottom of the heel, making it difficult to walk correctly. Treatment typically includes PRICEMM and pain medications (see Questions 10 and 11). Padding or protecting the injured area with a gel-based heel cup or donut pad can be helpful as well. If symptoms worsen, see your healthcare provider. He or she will examine your heel and may order X-rays, MRI, or other tests to rule out a fracture.

Plantar fasciitis is a result of microtears and inflammation in the plantar fascia, a tough, flat structure that helps form the arch of the foot. This may be due to an overuse injury (too much, too soon, too fast) or for no apparent reason at all. Pain is focused on the bottom of the heel and is typically worse with the first few steps in the morning (after sleeping all night) or after a prolonged period of time at rest. Jumping or pushing off also makes symptoms worse. Treatment includes stretching of the Achilles tendon and calf muscles (see **Figure 20** on page 202), ice massage (see Question 10), pain medications (see Question 11), gel-based heel cups, and perhaps night splints that keep the Achilles tendon and foot stretched. Arch supports may also help. If your symptoms do not improve with these measures, see your healthcare professional. He or she will examine your heel and may order X-rays or other tests. Your healthcare provider may also offer a corticosteroid injection for your injury (see Question 12). If your symptoms still do not improve, you may consider surgical treatments, but the postoperative recovery is very long. Discuss the risks and benefits of any of these treatments frankly with your provider.

Fat pad atrophy, also known as fat pad insufficiency and fat pad syndrome, occurs when the cushioning fat pad under your heel breaks down and thins out. This results in less cushioning between the floor and your heel, and consequently, heel pain. This can occur with repetitive pounding on the unprotected heel. Unfortunately, this problem is very difficult to treat. Gel-based heel cups, cushioned shoes, and other ways of relieving this stress are your best bet. If your symptoms worsen, see your healthcare provider. He or she will examine your heel and may order X-rays, MRI, or other tests to rule out a fracture.

76. My arches feel tired or sore after running. Now what?

The arches that help shape the undersurface (plantar surface) of our feet are very important. They help define the overall mechanics of how the foot moves and adapts to the ground surface on which we walk, run, jump, and play. They provide support and shock absorption. By doing so, our arches affect every other body part—from the rest of the foot, to the knees, hips, back, and neck. And when our plantar arches feel tired or sore, we should listen to them. The plantar arch is actually two arches in one: the longitudinal arch, and the transverse arch. Together they define the shape of the plantar arch. There are basically three types of plantar arches: normal (neutral), high (cavus), and flat (planus) arches. The definitions of the various types are controversial and complicated, but most people have arches that resemble one type more than the others to varying degrees.

When our arches are sore or tired from running, it is usually due to a mismatch between the shoes and inserts we may be wearing, the shape of our arch, and the demands of the sporting or exercise activity we are doing. Differences in weight, width, materials, sole designs, shapes, cushioning, and lacing patterns can make finding the right shoe perplexing. Brand names, looks, and the price tag contribute very little to nothing in regards to protecting your feet and preventing injury. Proper fit and overall design mean a whole lot more. Some useful tips in finding a shoe that fits well include:

Brand names, looks, and the price tag contribute very little to nothing in regards to protecting your feet and preventing injury.

- A good time to try on shoes is after working out or the end of the day, because our feet tend to swell.
- Make sure there is about one inch between your longest toe and the end of the shoe.
- Make sure your heel does not slip.
- Wear the same type of sock that you will be wearing with the shoes after you buy them.
- Walk, jog, or even run and jump in the shoes to try them out. Test run them with the actual activities that you will be using them for.
- The shoes should feel comfortable out of the box. Do not feel like you have break in the shoes to make them comfortable.
- If the shoe seems almost perfect, except for one small detail of fit, ask the store representative if they know of any lacing techniques that may help make the fit feel more like a custom fit.

Shoe manufacturers make shoes that cater not only to certain sports, but also to certain foot types. Specialty running stores are a good place to start looking for the right kind of shoe for your particular foot shape. Expect to spend 15–45 minutes working with the store staff in choosing the right shoe for you. Since everyone is unique, it is important to take a personalized approach to shoe wear. If you continue to have symptoms, see a healthcare professional familiar with sports medicine concerns. He or she will examine your feet and how you walk and may order an X-ray or other tests. Your healthcare provider will then make recommendations for your training practices and equipment, including shoes, or even orthotic inserts.

Also, athletic shoes, especially those used for running sports, wear out rather quickly. When they do so, they lose much of the protective and performance-enhancing properties they were designed to provide. The mileage or shelf life at which you should replace a shoe varies depending on the manufacturer and shoe model. However, a good guideline is to replace your running shoe after 2 years if you do not run regularly. If you do run regularly, replace your shoes every 6–12 months or every 300–600 miles, depending on your training habits and surfaces.

In general a high cavus arch has a lot of support, but very little cushioning and shock absorption. They also tend to roll in, putting you at risk for ankle injuries. Therefore, people with high arches may benefit from a more flexible, cushioned shoe, with a more semicurved sole, and perhaps a little extra lateral support. Certain types of cushioning and laterally wedged orthotic inserts may also be helpful; these are available over the counter or as custom-made orthotics from a healthcare provider, physical therapist, athletic trainer, or orthotist.

Flat planus arches are flexible and shock absorbing but lack support. They also tend to roll in. People with flatter arches may need more arch support in the form of orthotic inserts, and a more supportive, motion control shoe with medial arch support.

Neutral arches usually do well with many of the available running shoes today. However, if your arches feel tired or sore after running, your foot (and therefore your arch) may actually undergo some abnormal motion with stepping. This motion may explain why you still have symptoms despite having normal-looking arches. One of the most common types of abnormal motions is too much pronation. As we take a step, our feet naturally roll in as we shift weight onto them. They do so in such a direction as to bring the big-toe side of the foot down towards the ground. This is called pronation, and should occur at a certain speed, and only to a certain amount. In many runners with neutral arches, they pronate too much (hyperpronation), or they pronate too soon or too quickly (early pronation). These athletes may benefit from running shoes with a special type of foam in the sole, just under the arch. Many of these shoes are called stability shoes. There are also both over-the-counter and custom-made orthotic inserts that may help control this pronation as well.

In addition to shoe wear and orthotics, arch problems may also require specific rehabilitation exercises. Your healthcare provider may recommend working with a physical therapist familiar with foot problems to help maximize your foot health and performance.

PART SIX

Sport-Specific Injuries

What are the most common injuries in baseball, and how can I prevent them?

What is Little League elbow, and what should I do about it?

How can I make exercising in cold weather as safe as possible?

More . . .

77. What are the most common injuries in baseball, and how can I prevent them?

Baseball is still a very popular sport with active participants from childhood to adulthood. Injuries are usually overuse in nature, but unique traumatic injuries are also quite common. Injuries in younger baseball players are mostly to the head and face, whereas adults are more likely to suffer strains and sprains of the ankle and knee as well fractures of the nose and lower leg.

The most common overuse problem in baseball is the shoulder and elbow. Rotator cuff tendonitis (see Question 32) and shoulder instability (looseness) (see Question 34) predominate, as they do in swimming. Elbow issues may be Little League elbow as discussed in Question 78 or chronic strain of the ligaments or muscles on the inside part of the elbow (UCL strain and medial epicondylitis; see Question 38) in the older competitor. Shoulder and elbow problems may occur in all players, but are more commonly seen in pitchers. Treatment of these problems centers on periods of rest from the sport, strengthening, stretching, and working on throwing mechanics when returning to activity. Overall fitness is very important as mentioned earlier in this book. Throwing mechanics is not all related to shoulder and elbow strength. There is a **kinetic chain** from ground contact to the hand releasing the ball. Each component is important. Overall fitness, leg strength, hamstring flexibility, and core strength all contribute to the proper throw as well injury prevention.

Kinetic chain

A term coined by Ben Kibler identifying the series of joint motions to generate a sport or occupational joint motion.

Most injuries occur during game play rather than practice.

Traumatic injuries can come from being struck by a thrown or batted ball and from collisions with other players, equipment in the field or foul area, and with the bases with base running. Collisions with other players and its injury patterns are more common in adults, and being struck by a bat is more common in children. Most injuries occur during game play rather than practice. Sliding injuries may cause significant skin abrasions as well as hand and foot injuries when sliding incorrectly into a fixed base.

Facial injuries are usually traumatic from collisions and being struck by a ball and may include facial and jaw fractures and eye and dental injuries (see Questions 24, 25, and 26). In the upper extremity, overuse shoulder injuries from repetitive throwing, inside elbow pain (golfer's elbow), and hand injuries with finger fractures and mallet finger (see Question 45) are most common. Lower extremity injuries include knee sprains, abrasions from sliding, and ankle injuries (see Question 72). Achilles tendon rupture (see Question 74) is a common injury in older adult leagues when running the bases.

Commotio cordis is a cardiac condition unique to the child baseball player. When a child is struck directly in the chest by a ball at a certain moment in the cardiac cycle, a cardiac arrest can ensue. This is extremely rare, because the impact has to be at a precise moment in the electrical cycle of the heart. Studies to look at the use of softer balls or chest protectors have been done, but they have not been found to be effective. The best management is to be aware that this condition exists and to have appropriate equipment or resources on site. This includes an automated external defibrillator (AED) or emergency medical services (EMS)—an ambulance for games.

Due to all of the aforementioned, there are recommended safety tips for safe baseball and softball play. In particular for adults, a good preseason conditioning program with stretching and strengthening (especially for the rotator cuff in pitchers) as well as pregame and prepractice stretching and warm-up will prevent many overuse conditions. Monitor and limit the number of pitches for all pitchers, but in particular for children (see Question 78). Batters should wear an approved batting helmet with double ear covers and should consider a facial protector. Catchers should have properly fitting gear with shin guards, chest protector, mask, and helmet.

In the field, the use of breakaway bases; padded fences, walls, and posts; and adequate protection for players in the dugout are all good safety measures. Instruct players, in particular youth players, on proper sliding techniques. Finally, injured players should undergo a proper rehabilitation program and be ready to play prior to attempting to return.

78. What is Little League elbow, and what should I do about it?

Little League elbow is a diagnosis that identifies a collection of several elbow problems in youth throwers. Often associated with pitchers, who do more throwing, it may be seen in any youth baseball players. Next to shoulder pain, elbow pain is the most common problem in youth pitchers. Mechanically the valgus load defines a bending moment on the arm moving the hand away from the body. These valgus loads stretch the structures on the inside of the elbow and compress the structures on the outside. Due to this stress, there is a collection of diagnoses of inside elbow apophysitis, stretching of the inside ligaments (the medial collateral ligaments), bony injury to the outside part of the elbow joint (capitellar osteochondral injuries), and stress fracture of the olecranon (the bony part of the back of the elbow). When a pitcher complains of elbow pain it should prompt an assessment of his overall throwing stress and mechanics as well; he should be evaluated with a physician familiar with youth elbow problems.

Contributing factors to the development of symptoms include age, increased weight, decreased height, lifting weights during the season, playing baseball in addition to the team's league games, decreased self-satisfaction, arm fatigue during a game and throwing more that 600 pitches in a season. Pitchers throwing breaking balls (curveballs and sliders) are more likely to complain of arm pain. Throwing curveballs has been associated with a 50% increase in shoulder pain while sliders may significantly increase the risk of elbow complaints.

The USA Baseball Medical and Safety Advisory Committee has made the following recommendations in a position statement addressing youth baseball injuries. Recommended pitch counts by age are:

8–10 years, 50 per game, 1000 pitches per season, and 2000 per year

11–12 years, 75 per game, 1000 per season, and 3000 per year

13–14 years, 75 per game, 1000 per season, and 3000 per year

15–16 years, 90 per game and 3000 per year

17–18 years, 105 per game

Pitchers should not compete for more than 9 months per year and should avoid overhead activities during the 3-month off-season. Pitchers should be removed from the game when they experience fatigue and should not return to pitching in the same game. Pitchers should be encouraged to learn the change-up pitch as opposed to curve balls and sliders. The average age recommendation for learning new types of pitches include: fastball, 8; change-up, 10; curveball, 14; knuckleball, 15; slider, 16; forkball, 16; splitter, 16; screwball, 17.

Pitchers should be encouraged to learn the change-up pitch as opposed to curve balls and sliders.

Additionally, coaches should monitor pitchers' activity outside of team play and practice to look for other contributing stresses to a pitcher's shoulder such as weight lifting and out-of-league play.

79. What is Little League shoulder, and what should I do about it?

After the elbow, the shoulder is the most commonly stressed joint in the body. The mechanics of the baseball throw impart stresses on the elbow and shoulder in all phases of the throw.

Throwing athletes often develop shoulder problems related to instability (loose shoulder) and sports-induced weakness of the rotator cuff and scapular stabilizing muscles. Range of motion problems or loss of motion is uncommon in younger athletes and stretching activities are generally not necessary other than in the context of warming up for activity. Rotator cuff-specific training prior to injury should be performed in addition to a general resistance exercise program that will focus more on larger power muscles and core strengthening.

Rotator cuff strengthening exercises focus on the strength of the supraspinatus and external rotators of the shoulder. Exercises should be performed to a count of 6 (2 seconds for contraction and 4 seconds negative) with 3- to 5-pound weights.

Scapular stabilizers

The muscles around the shoulder blade that support the shoulder blade when the arm and shoulder is moved through its wide range of motion.

Scapular stabilizers are those muscles around the shoulder blade that support and position the shoulder blade during overhead activities. They include the levator scapula and trapezius that elevate the scapula, the rhomboids that help retract the scapula, and the serratus anterior and posterior that helps with retraction and keeping the scapula on the chest wall during sport-specific motions. Exercises generally involve shoulder elevation, retraction, and pinching the shoulder blades together. These should be performed with lighter weights (3–5 pounds) at 6 seconds per repetition.

Kinetic chain

A term coined by Ben Kibler identifying the series of joint motions to generate a sport or occupational joint motion.

Finally, we cannot overemphasize the importance of proper throwing mechanics and attention to the other important body portions of the kinetic chain. The **kinetic chain** is a term coin by Dr. Ben Kibler to identify the total body motion required to perform an athletic maneuver. Almost all athletic maneuvers start with ground contact and transmit energy from that contact to the final contact with the ball or racket. In baseball, this means that shoulder problems should also lead to evaluation and treatment of core strengthening, hamstring flexibility, and lower extremity strengthening as well as the elbow, shoulder, and upper back exercises. Addressing all these issues is important.

80. What are the most common running injuries, and how can I prevent them?

The most common injuries associated with running sports include:

- Patellofemoral pain syndrome, patellar tendonitis, and quadriceps tendonitis (see Question 62)
- Overtraining (see Question 15)
- Groin strain, Gilmore's groin, and snapping hip or Trochanteric Bursitis (see Questions 56–59)
- Hamstring strains (see Question 60)
- Snapping knee (ITB) syndrome (see Question 66)
- Shin splints and stress fractures (see Questions 69 and 70)
- Calf strains and Achilles tendon problems (see Questions 71 and 74)
- Heel problems and problems affecting the plantar arches (see Questions 75 and 76)
- Skin blisters (see Question 14)

For specific information regarding each of the aforementioned conditions, please see the corresponding question and answer, referenced in the list. Overall, most running injuries are a result of improper warm-up, lack of regular stretching, and overuse problems (doing too much, too soon, too fast). To prevent running injuries, it is important to stretch regularly, especially the calf, hamstring, and quadriceps muscles. Prevent overuse problems by gradually introducing changes in training habits, intensity, equipment, surfaces, and nutrition. Do not increase running mileage more than 10% per week. Maintain adequate caloric intake, and train with appropriate hydration and nutrition practices that mimic the conditions likely encountered in any sporting event in which you may be participating. Finally, make sure you choose the right running shoes for your specific sporting activity, environment, and body (see Question 76), and do not forget to replace them regularly. Additionally, it is important to select training clothing, accessories, and apparel that fit the environmental conditions in which you train and compete. This is especially important in cold and hot weather conditions (see Questions 83 and 84).

81. What are the most common basketball injuries, and how can I prevent them?

The most common injuries associated with basketball include:

- Ankle sprains (see Question 72)
- Patellofemoral pain syndrome, patellar tendonitis, quadriceps tendonitis (see Question 62)
- Shin splints and stress fractures (see Questions 69 and 70)
- Calf strains and Achilles tendon problems (see Questions 71 and 74)
- Heel problems and problems affecting the plantar arches (Questions 75 and 76)
- Skin blisters (see Question 14)
- ACL injuries (see Questions 1 and 64)
- Concussions and other head injuries (see Question 21)
- Facial, jaw, eye, and nose injuries (see Questions 24 through 26)
- Loose, broken, or knocked-out teeth (see Question 28)
- Scrapes, cuts, chafing, and road rash (see Question 13)
- Hand and wrist injuries, especially finger injuries (see Questions 41 through 47)

For specific information regarding each of the aforementioned conditions, please see the corresponding question and answer as referenced. It is important to stretch regularly, especially the calf, hamstring, and quadriceps muscles. Prevent overuse problems by gradually introducing changes in training habits, intensity, equipment, surfaces, and nutrition. Maintain adequate caloric intake, and train with appropriate hydration and nutrition practices that mimic the conditions likely to be encountered in any sporting event in which you may be participating. Many athletes use ankle bracing and taping techniques and wear high-top shoes to prevent ankle sprains. The best way to prevent ankle sprains, however, is to strengthen and train the muscles that support and stabilize the ankle during various maneuvers used in basketball. For the other conditions, please see their corresponding sections.

82. What are the most common skiing and snowboarding injuries, and how can I prevent them?

The most common injuries associated with skiing and snowboarding include:

- MCL sprains (see Question 63)
- ACL injuries (see Questions 1 and 64)
- Hand and wrist injuries, especially finger injuries (see Questions 41 through 47)
- Thumb injuries, especially ulnar collateral ligament sprains (also known as skier's thumb) (see Question 44)
- Ankle sprains (see Question 72)
- Proximal tibial fractures, including tibial plateau fractures
- Shoulder injuries (see Questions 32 through 34)
- Concussions and other head injuries (see Question 21)
- Nosebleeds and facial injuries (see Questions 23 and 24)
- Neck injuries, including burners or stingers (see Question 29 through 31)
- Injuries to the chest, back, and trunk (see Questions 48 through 53)
- Cold temperature injuries (see Question 83)
- Altitude illness

For specific information regarding each of the aforementioned conditions, please see the corresponding question and answer. In general, proper preseason conditioning may help prevent injuries. This includes quadriceps, hamstring, calf, core, and neck stretching, strengthening, and endurance training (see the corresponding body part sections for details). Knee injuries seen in skiing may be decreased with newer designs in binding and boot designs that allow the skis to break away as the skier falls and tumbles. Proper binding adjustment and daily self-testing of the bindings ensure that they are functioning appropriately. Goggles and other protective eyewear are essential. But these advances in equipment technology alone are not enough. Avoid skiing when more than moderately fatigued, and always use good skiing technique. Ask a ski instruction professional for details in good skiing technique. Helmets, wrist protective devices, boots with stiff inner linings, elbow and knee pads, and protective eyewear are recommended for snowboarders. Good technique and equipment safety are also important for snowboarders.

Altitude sickness and other altitude-related conditions may present with headache, dizziness, nausea, and irritability. Skiers and snowboarders with more severe cases may develop confusion, trouble breathing, unstable vital signs, and even coma. These can lead to an emergent, life-threatening condition, so seek medical attention as soon as possible. Part of the treatment of altitude sickness is to decrease the altitude and rest. Prevent altitude sickness by ascending to altitude gradually. Spend at least 2 nights getting used to the increased altitude for every 2000 feet you climb over 8000 feet. Avoid immediately climbing to greater than 10,000 feet, and monitor how you feel closely. There are also prescription medications that can be used to help prevent altitude illnesses. See your healthcare professional if you are planning to use medications to prevent altitude sickness.

83. How can I make exercising in cold weather as safe as possible?

Cold injuries include hypothermia and frostbite. Hypothermia occurs when the core body temperature of the athlete drops and the athlete is unable to raise the temperature. This can lead to many types of problems in the body. In mild cases, the hypothermic athlete can develop confusion, slurred speech, amnesia, fast heart rate, fast breathing, and shivering. More significant hypothermia can result in lethargy, hallucinations, coma, decreased heart rate and breathing, and joint rigidity. Prevent hypothermia while you exercise by increasing the heat your body makes and decreasing how much heat your body loses. Frequent meals and snacks, adequate fluid intake, and staying active all help to generate heat. Using versatile, layered, cold-weather clothing with a good balance between insulation and breathability helps trap and prevent the loss of heat. Water-repellant shells, windproof layers, and ventilation ports are a plus. Maintain adequate trunk warmth, and prevent heat loss from the head and face using a hat, hood, or balaclava. The goal is to layer in such a way that you stay warm, without being excessively warm or sweaty with the activity you intend to do. Many specialty outdoor-sports store employees participate in cold weather sports. They can be very helpful, so feel free to ask them or more experienced athletes what they recommend. Do not forget to warm up and stretch appropriately before exercising in the cold.

Frostbite is a localized freezing of the tissues on exposed areas, such as the hands, feet, face, and ears. The best way to prevent frostbite is to cover these areas and to keep them warm. So-called cold protecting ointments and emollients generally do not work to prevent frostbite, and in fact, may actually make it more likely. The best prevention is simply to limit direct exposure of the skin to the cold.

The goal is to layer in such a way that you stay warm, without being excessively warm or sweaty with the activity you intend to do.

84. How can I make exercising in hot and humid weather as safe as possible?

Exercise-related heat injuries include heat cramps, heat exhaustion, and heatstroke. These occur when the athlete has generated or retained too much heat and is unable to shed the heat fast enough, raising the core body temperature and leading to all sorts of problems. Mild cases of heat injury result in muscle cramps, while cases of heat exhaustion present with fatigue, weakness, dizziness, headaches, poor coordination, confusion, and irritability. This can lead to the athlete being unable to continue the exercise activity and may even progress to heatstroke, a life-threatening condition with more profound confusion, coma, and problems with the heart and kidneys, as well as muscle breakdown. It is therefore most important to prevent heat injuries. To do this, take the following measures when considering whether to exercise in hot environments:

- If possible, avoid training in the hottest and most humid of environments. If available, a device called a wet bulb globe can be used to determine how safe the environment is for exercise. In general, avoid wet bulb globe temperatures greater than 28°C.
- Consider training during early morning or late evening hours, in order to avoid exercising during the hottest and most humid times of the day.
- Gradually build a tolerance to hot and humid environments. Start with limiting your exposure to the environment to 30–60 minutes a day, and increase gradually based on how you feel.
- Wear appropriate, loose, cool, and lightweight clothing. Consider a moisture-wicking type of garment, designed to help sweat evaporate and keep you cool. Check with more experienced athletes or the sales staff at specialty outdoor-sports stores to find the right kind of apparel for your desired activities.

- Maintain good hydration. Water is good, but make sure you include fluids that include electrolytes. Drink frequently before, during, and after exercise. If you feel thirsty, you have already been dehydrated.
- Working on increasing muscle conditioning and endurance may prevent heat cramps.

85. What are the most common bicycling injuries, and how can I prevent them?

The most common injuries associated with cycling include:

- Concussions and other head injuries (see Question 21)
- Neck injuries, including burners or stingers (see Questions 29 through 31)
- Back pain (see Questions 51 through 53)
- Scrapes, cuts, chafing, and road rash (see Question 13)
- Skin blisters (see Question 14)
- Overtraining (see Question 15)
- Iliotialband Friction Syndrome of the knee (see Question 59)
- Patellofemoral pain syndrome, patellar tendonitis, and quadriceps tendonitis (see Question 62)
- Stress fractures (see Questions 69 and 70)
- Achilles tendon problems (see Question 74)
- Heel problems and problems affecting the plantar arches (Questions 75 and 76)
- Pudendal neuropathy, trauma to genitalia, and impotence
- Saddle sores
- Shoulder injuries (see Questions 32 through 34)
- **Handlebar palsy** (ulnar neuropathy) (Question 40)
- Wrist injuries (see Question 41)

Handlebar palsy

Injury to the ulnar nerve in the palm caused by a bicycle's handlebar.

Injuries associated with various cycling sports can be divided into 1) injuries related to falls and collisions, 2) other acute injuries, and 3) overuse injuries. For specific information regarding each of the aforementioned conditions, please see the corresponding question and answer. It is important to stretch regularly, especially the calf, hamstring, and quadriceps muscles. Prevent overuse problems by gradually introducing changes in training habits, intensity, equipment, and nutrition. Maintain adequate caloric intake, and train with appropriate hydration and nutrition practices that mimic the conditions likely encountered in any sporting event in which you may be participating. Many falls and collisions, as well as overuse injuries, can be prevented with appropriate equipment fitting, use, and modifications. It is extremely important for cycling athletes to use a bicycle well fitted to the rider, and well suited for the demands of the activity intended (see Question 86).

86. What should I look for in my biking equipment to prevent injuries?

Many cycling injuries can be prevented with appropriate equipment fitting, use, and modifications. Do not underestimate how much the right equipment can both protect you from injury and boost your performance and therefore enhance your enjoyment of the activity.

A properly fitted, protective helmet is an absolute must for all cyclists. Ensure that the helmet is snug, level, stable, and not overly tight. The helmet should not give you a headache or make you dizzy, but it should also not move excessively on your head. Avoid wearing a hat or bandana between the helmet and your head, as this may cause unwanted motion. Make sure the helmet is level, with the front just above your eyebrows (or glasses). If you walk into a wall with your helmet on, the helmet should hit the wall before your nose does. Adjust the chin strap and use fit pads to ensure a secure, stable, level, yet comfortable fit. Make sure that you can barely see the front rim of the helmet when you wear it. The Y on each of the side straps should sit just below your ears. The chin strap should be tight enough, so that opening you mouth very widely pulls down on the helmet a little (but should not cause discomfort). A good way to test how securely fit your helmet is is to strap your helmet on, and push or slap the secured helmet firmly at various angles; it should move less than an inch.

Wear the proper clothing to protect yourself from the environment (see Questions 83 and 84). Padded gloves designed to protect your palms may help prevent ulnar nerve problems. Padded shorts help make riding more comfortable and may help prevent saddle sores and other saddle-related problems. Certain apparel safety features may be important for certain types of riding. For example, in addition to more robust helmets, extreme downhill mountain biking may require clothing with protective pads and plates, and special gloves designed for that type of activity. Check with experienced athletes or the sales staff at specialty cycling stores to find the right apparel and safety equipment for your desired activities.

See and be seen. Protective eyewear protects the eyes from debris and sun glare. If you will be riding in decreased lighting, reflective tape, safety lights, and a headlight (or headlamp) are a must for safe biking.

There are several saddle designs available that include a cut-out or low-density foam section in the center. This takes the pressure off of the pubic bone and nearby nerves, and may prevent nerve problems in the seated area, impotence, and trauma to the genitals.

It is extremely important for cycling athletes to use a bicycle that is well fitted to the rider, and well suited for the demands of the activity intended. There several different types of bicycles, including various materials and overall frame design shapes and fork designs, as well as the types of accompanying equipment and other accessories. These include road (racing) bikes, mountain (all-terrain) bikes, triathlon bikes, time-trial bikes, touring bikes, city (cruiser) bikes, and hybrid bikes. Check with experienced athletes or the sales staff at specialty cycling stores to find the right type of bike for your desired activities.

It is also important to have a bike with size and dimensions that fit your body and riding style. There are many commercially available bicycle measuring systems (for a fee) to accomplish this. These are often used by specialty cycling stores that cater to the serious or competitive rider. However, you can perform your own fitting by addressing the following six basic adjustments: 1) frame size, 2) seat height, 3) saddle position, 4) saddle angle, 5) handlebar height, and 6) handlebar reach. In general, the guidelines that follow are not absolute rules. They are a good place to start, and you should adjust these parameters to comfort as you become more familiar with your bike. Make only one minor adjustment at a time.

1. To find the optimal frame size, straddle the bike frame with your feet on the ground. For a road bike, there should be 1–2 inches between your crotch and the top of the frame, and for a mountain bike, there should be 3–4 inches.

2. For a good estimate of the right seat height, sit on the bike with your heels in the pedals, using a nearby wall for balance. Place the pedals in the 6 and 12 o'clock positions. Adjust the seat height so that the knee corresponding to the lower pedal is straight. After subsequent rides, you may make further adjustments to the seat height.

3. For the right saddle position, sit on the bike with your feet in the pedals, using a nearby wall for balance. Place the pedals in the 3 and 9 o'clock positions. Adjust the saddle position until a straight, up-and-down, plumb line can be drawn from the edge of the front knee to the axle of the front pedal.

4. As for the saddle angle, make sure you adjust the angle so that you can actually sit *on* the saddle—with your pelvis level—and not angled downward in the front (causing a tendency to slide forward). For most saddles, the nose (front) of the saddle should be slightly higher than the rear.

5. Handlebar height depends on what type of riding you will be doing. The most important thing is that you are comfortable. Road and mountain bikers generally prefer a handlebar height 2–3 inches below the saddle height, while touring bikers like it at the same height as the saddle. A good rule of thumb is to choose the lowest handlebar height where you can still feel completely comfortable.

6. As far as handlebar reach (distance) is concerned, consider starting with one that places your elbows at 90° angles and adjust from there to comfort.

87. What are the most common soccer injuries, and how can I prevent them?

It is estimated that here are 40 million participants in soccer worldwide. It is the most popular sport in the world. There are an estimated 200,000 youth (under 15) injuries per year in this sport. Most of these injuries can be prevented with the proper wear of safety gear and following the rules of play. Older players sustain more severe injuries and girls tend to be injured more often than boys. Injury rates are about 1% under age 12 and 8% in high school. Most injuries are caused by illegal play, poor field conditions, or incorrect heading.

Most injuries are sprains and strains; of these, the most common are ankle injuries, followed by knee injuries. Of these acute injuries, the ankle sprain (see Question 72) is most common, and in the knee, sprains of the MCL or ACL (see Questions 63 and 64) and meniscal (knee cartilage) injuries (see Question 67) are common. Overuse injuries in youth players include Sever's disease, Osgood-Schlatter disease, patellofemoral pain, shin splints, and stress fractures of the leg (see Questions 19, 62, 69, and 70). Upper extremity injuries are related to collisions or falls, and acromioclavicular strains (AC separation; see Question 33), contusions, and wrist injuries (see Question 41) are common. Head injuries (see Question 21) are rare and are associated with aggressive play and head-on-head contact or contact with the goal post. Contact with the goal post is associated with more severe injuries often resulting in an emergency room evaluation.

Injuries can be prevented if players wear shin guards, adequately warm up, and follow the rules of play. Soccer goals should be affixed to the ground properly and children should not hang on the crossbar. Injuries have been associated with tipping movable goals. Padding of goal posts will also reduce more severe injuries associated with collisions with the post. Sliding tackles from behind are illegal and coaches should insist that players adhere to safe play rules.

The issue of children heading the ball is controversial. There have been several recent scientific studies looking at changes in brain function after a session of heading the ball. Although there is no clear evidence that there is a long-term or short-term decline in brain function, there are often complaints of nausea or headaches. It is also clear that there is a skill to heading to minimize the effects on the brain after heading. For this reason, children should have a certain amount of skill, neck strength, and supervised practice of heading before they should head in competition. This is likely not going to occur under the age of 12, but there is no set age recommendation.

88. What are the most common football, lacrosse, and rugby injuries, and how can I prevent them?

Football, rugby, and soccer have similar roots, with football being born form rugby and rugby from soccer with a famous play at a soccer game at Rugby College in England in 1825. American football has close to 3 million participants at all levels in the United States. Rugby is played worldwide and is gaining popularity in the United States. Lacrosse is predominantly a U.S. sport played mostly at the high school and college level, with some adult leagues. There are an estimated 250,000–300,000 lacrosse players nationwide with a 4:1 ratio of male to female players. Football and rugby are more similar and lacrosse is more closely related to hockey in its play and injury patterns.

In 1995, the National Electronic Injury Surveillance System reported nearly 390,000 football injuries requiring an emergency room visit. Of these injuries, 33% were sprains and strains, 24% fractures (broken bones), and 17% bruises and abrasions. Concussions accounted for 1.6% of the injuries. One state database for high school football reported a single-season injury rate of 39% for varsity players. The most frequently injured body parts were the hip, leg, or thigh (17.3%); the forearm, wrist, or hand (15%); the knee (14.5%), and the ankle or foot (14.2%). Head, neck, and spine injuries accounted for 11.3% of the injuries. Injury patterns are similar in lacrosse, with the added injury source from being struck by the thrown ball or the opponent's stick.

Common injuries in these sports by body area are:

- Head—concussion, eye injuries, lacerations, and cauliflower ear (in rugby) (see Questions 21, 24, 25, and 27)
- Neck—sprain, stinger/burner, neck fractures (see Questions 29 through 31)
- Shoulder—AC sprain, dislocation, and clavicle fracture (see Questions 33 and 34)
- Elbow—dislocation
- Wrist—sprain, fractures (see Question 41)
- Hand—finger dislocation and fractures (see Questions 44 and 45)
- Back—sprain, spondylolysis (see Questions 18 and 51)
- Hip—contusion
- Knee—MCL and ACL tear, meniscal injury, and patellar dislocation (see Questions 62 through 65)

- Ankle—sprain and fractures (see Question 72)
- Foot—**Lisfranc joint** (midfoot) sprain and fractures, and **turf toe**

Lisfranc joint

The collection of the joints in the middle portion of the foot between the tarsal and metatarsal joints approximately in the middle portion of the arch.

Turf toe

Injury to the big toe when it is hyperextended, often on artificial turf, injuring the ball joint of the big toe.

Injury is inherent with such high-demand contact sports, but the athlete brings characteristics that may predispose himself or herself to injury, which, if addressed, may prevent injury. All athletes should undergo a preparticipation physical examination (PPE) in accordance with the guidelines put forth in the PPE monograph endorsed by the AAFP-American Academy of Family Practice; AAP-American Academy of Pediatrics; ACSM-American College of Sports Medicine; AMSSM-American Medical Society of Sports Medicine; AOSSM-American Orthopedic Society of Sports Medicine. This assessment includes a review of medical history and a good cardiac and musculoskeletal assessment. Athletes should be of appropriate maturity and physical development to follow rules and learn skills.

Preseason conditioning and strength training should focus on endurance, overall muscular strength, and neck and shoulder strength.

Preseason conditioning and strength training should focus on endurance, overall muscular strength, and neck and shoulder strength. Equipment should be properly fitted to include a helmet with an appropriate face mask, shoulder pads, knee and hip guards, mouth guard, and shoes.

89. What are the most common swimming and diving injuries, and how can I prevent them?

Swimming is an excellent low-impact sport activity enjoyed by athletes of all ages. For most competitive athletes, swimming is a year-round sport with no down time. This can be concerning because of the risk of injury and overtraining. Most injuries in swimming are overuse in nature and the most commonly injured body area or joint is the shoulder. As many as 50–75% of swimmers at various ages have problems with shoulder pain.

The four primary strokes in swimming (freestyle, breaststroke, butterfly, and backstroke) each result in their own injury patterns based on the stroke mechanics and their demands on the body. Poor stroke mechanics, overuse, weakness, and overtraining are often the underlying causes of the various injuries seen in this sport. Freestyle injuries are generally limited to the shoulder. The butterfly stroke may also generate shoulder overuse problems, but also tendonitis in the foot, lower back problems (spondylolysis) and patellofemoral pain. The backstroke is probably the most stressful stroke on the shoulder, and with poor turns, it may be associated with head injuries from contact with the wall. The breaststroke additionally stresses the shoulder, but it can also cause hip and knee problems. One unique injury of the knee called breaststroker's knee is a chronic strain of the medial collateral ligament (MCL) of the knee. Independent of the stroke itself, the year-round participation, long hours in the water, and sleep deprevation from early morning workouts before school, overtraining is a common problem in the more competitive athletes. See Question 15 for more discussion.

Shoulder problems predominate in swimming. For most swimmers, instability or looseness of the shoulder and weakness of the rotator cuff muscles are common (see Questions 32 and 34). There is argument as to whether the sport participation causes shoulder looseness or if athletes with loose shoulders tend to gravitate toward this sport. The number one treatment and prevention strategy is proper stroke mechanics and rotator cuff rehabilitative exercises. These exercises are demonstrated in **Figures 2 and 3**.

Diving is a competitive sport with participants at the high school, collegiate, and international levels. In many respects diving is like gymnastics on the platform or spring board, and many divers are ex-gymnasts. Most injuries in diving are associated with poor technique with the diver striking the board or platform on the descent or with problems upon entering the water. These injuries may include those associated with diving in shallow water or poor entry technique with dives from greater heights. Prevention of dive injuries is best approached with proper supervision of practice sessions as well instruction of the dive technique.

Ultimately treatment of these underlying problems includes appropriate rehabilitation and proper stroke mechanics or dive technique as the athlete or individual resumes participation.

90. What is swimmer's ear, and what should I do about it?

Swimmer's ear is an infection of the external canals of the ear. It is universally seen in aquatic athletes. When you are submerged in water, water may become trapped in the external canal. In most cases, this drains on its own over the first few hours after you are out of the water.

In some people, the water remains and changes the chemical mix of the canal. Bacteria are not uncommon in the ear canal, but they are kept in check by an acidic environment in the external canal. When water is trapped, the acidity changes and bacteria and fungal elements are provided with a wet environment to foster overgrowth.

Symptoms of swimmer's ear include whitish drainage, pain (especially when the ear lobe is tugged), and decreased hearing. The pain may be so severe that even talking and chewing may aggravate symptoms.

Treatments may include prescription antibiotic ear drops or even home remedy treatments and then a prevention program. Most doctors will prescribe some kind of antibiotic ear drop to be used two to three times per day for a week. Athletes should use ear plugs or avoid submersion in the water while they are symptomatic. Home remedies could include the use of over-the-counter solutions e.g., acetic acid and aluminum acetate otic or making a home solution. You can make a home solution by mixing equal parts white vinegar with rubbing alcohol. Instill two drops of the solution into the ear three times daily for 3–5 days early in the course.

Prevention strategies include the use of ear plugs or placing acetic acid and aluminum acetate otic or the homemade solution in each ear after getting out of the water.

91. What are the most common golfing injuries, and how can I prevent them?

With the popularity of Tiger Woods and the worldwide explosion of golf participation, we are seeing more and more acute and chronic overuse injuries with golf. It is estimated that 18–20 million amateurs participate in golf in some fashion.

Most acute and chronic golf-related injuries involve the upper extremity and lower back. Low back pain tops them all and is likely related to poor fitness and poor swing mechanics (see Question 51). Treatment and prevention of low back pain include proper warm-up prior to practice and play, a program of core strengthening, and proper swing mechanics. All golfers want to hit the ball farther, but many have poor energy transfer and their swing overloads their lower backs. Taking lessons should be a cornerstone of treating back pain in a golfer.

In the upper extremity, shoulder injuries (rotator cuff tendonitis, see Question 32) are the most common, followed by elbow (see Question 38), wrist (see Question 41), and hand injuries. In the hand, trigger finger (see Question 47) is common and hook of the hamate injury is unique to golf. Shoulder, elbow, and trigger finger issues have been previously discussed. The hamate is a wrist bone on the ulnar side of the palm (side nearest the little finger). The hook of the hamate is a bony projection in the outside base of the palm. When a golfer is holding the golf club, the club rests on the hamate and the overlying soft tissues. When a golfer takes a large divot or hits a tree root while in or near the woods, the acute torque on the club can break the hook. This will present as local pain and swelling. It might not always be immediately obvious, but the pain will persist and limit ability to hold the club and make ball contact.

Safety issues in golf mainly focus on golf cart and lightning safety. Most injuries with golf cart use are associated with catching feet or hands that are hanging outside the cart and carts rolling over on hills. Simply paying attention to where you are and keeping your hands and feet inside the cart will avoid these very avoidable traumatic injuries. Despite continued attention to public awareness of lightning safety, this continues to be a problem. The problem is that most golf courses have wide open spaces and trees and golfers travel around holding a bag of 14 lightning rods called golf clubs. Lightening safety tips include:

1. Seek shelter at the first sign of a thunderstorm or lightning, especially if the course sounds a warning.
2. Do not stand under a tree in a lightning storm. Many courses have lightning-safe shelters throughout the course.
3. Stay away from your golf clubs.
4. If you still have metal spikes, take your shoes off.
5. Stay away from water.
6. Move away from your golf cart.
7. If you are in the open, get to a low place like a ravine or valley, or, if you cannot do that, crouch as close to the ground as you can with your head tucked down.

92. What are the most common tennis injuries, and how can I prevent them?

Tennis is an extraordinarily popular sport that is enjoyed by players of all ages. According to the United States Tennis Association (USTA), almost 25 million Americans played tennis in 2005. Men accounted for 52% of tennis players older than 6 years old, and the mean age of tennis players playing more than 21 times that year was 32. Among professional tennis players, 50–90% report injury in a 1-year time period, most of which were back, elbow, and shoulder injuries.

Tennis players commonly suffer injuries to both the upper and lower extremities. Lower extremity injuries encompass the gamut of injuries experienced by runners and soccer players, including ankle sprains (see Question 72), shin splints (see Question 69), calf strain and Achilles tendon injuries (see Questions 71 and 74), meniscus and ligamentous injuries of the knee (see Question 62 and 67), and groin injuries (see Question 56). As with any sport, an appropriate flexibility and strength training program coupled with appropriate warm-up, shoe wear, and equipment should be utilized to minimize injuries.

Upper extremity injuries in tennis players are more commonly attributed to overuse than a single traumatic injury, and most commonly include medial (inner) and lateral (outer) elbow injuries (see Questions 37 and 38), rotator cuff tendonitis and shoulder instability (see Questions 32 and 34), and back injuries (see Question 51). Overuse from repetitive ground strokes is commonly a cause of elbow injuries, while overhead strokes and serves, while they may also stress the elbow, tend to be more stressful to the shoulder and back. Pain in the lateral elbow is most commonly caused by irritation to the origin of the muscles involved in wrist extension and is known as lateral epicondylitis, or tennis elbow. These muscles are most commonly used in performing a backhand. Poor backhand form is commonly a factor in those who develop tennis elbow, and should be examined. Power from an appropriate one- or two-handed backhand comes from trunk rotation and weight transfer. In late strikers, or those who use the forearm and wrist to generate power, there is overuse of the muscles responsible for wrist extension.

Poor backhand form is commonly a factor in those who develop tennis elbow, and should be examined.

Medial elbow pain, also known as medial epicondylitis, or golfer's elbow (see Question 38) is most commonly associated with irritation of the origin of the muscles used in wrist flexion. Even a mechanically sound serve or overhead swing is quite taxing on this muscle group. Poor forehand mechanics can contribute to golfer's elbow. Late strikers or those who rely on wrist snap to generate force are more prone to straining the involved muscle group. The wrist should be held firmly in a neutral, rather than flexed position when striking the ball.

Prevention of elbow injuries is multifaceted. Careful attention must be paid to stroke mechanics and string tension should not be set too high. A tightly strung racket with synthetic stringing may impart more force to the involved muscles, as does off-center impact. Using a ball machine or striking the ball against a fixed wall typically increases repetitions dramatically and may incite or exacerbate an episode. Take care to build intensity and duration of activity slowly through a gradated program. Intensity, duration, and frequency of exercise should all be considered. Counterforce braces (see Question 37) may be applied to the forearm to change force distribution during activity only, and can be purchased at quality sporting goods stores. It was previously thought that improper grip size contributes to medial and lateral epicondylitis; however, more recent data suggests that this is not so.

Tennis, particularly serving and overhead strokes, imparts significant stress that may be injurious to the shoulder and back. Serving in particular is stressful when the arm rapidly accelerates from a fully abducted, externally rotated—or back scratch—position. Rotator cuff injuries are common, as is exacerbation of AC injury. Common symptoms include pain in the anterior shoulder, pain with elevation of the arm, and pain when reaching behind the back from above. Back injuries are consistent with those commonly incurred from flexion and twisting, which is to say they include disk herniation, muscular strain, and ligamentous sprain. Pain may be worse with sitting and improved with standing.

Prevention of all these injuries is similar in their goals and principles. Alterations may be made in the frequency, intensity, or duration of activity and a slow increase in activity is appropriate. Attention should be paid to stroke mechanics and to ensure that appropriate equipment is being used, particularly with regard to string tension. A preventive strengthening program for the rotator cuff (see Question 32) may be undertaken, and this should include scapular stabilization exercises. Back injuries may be less frequent with similar attention to stroke mechanics, and particularly to a core strengthening program (see Question 55).

93. What are the most common hockey injuries, and how can I prevent them?

Ice hockey is an extraordinarily fast-paced and aggressive collision sport that has many unique properties that increase the potential for injury. Professional hockey players skate at speeds of up to 30 mph on a hard ice surface, body check each other with wooden sticks, and send a vulcanized rubber puck that weighs 5.5 to 6 ounces traveling along the ice or through the air at up to 120 mph. Injury may be sustained from skating, falling, being struck by the puck or a stick, ice, goal posts, boards, and collisions with opposing players. Fighting is a controversial part of hockey culture and is considered more common in hockey than in most sports.

Hockey injuries have been studied extensively and acute injuries seem to make up about 85% of all injuries, and overuse pathology the remaining 15%. Injuries are more common during games than practice, and they increase in frequency with increasing age until peaking in late adolescence and early adulthood (17–19 years). Fatigue is a risk factor for injury, and protective equipment is critical to reducing injury frequency.

Because of the frequency of collisions and the number of injuries from the puck, skates, and stick, protective equipment plays a critical role in reducing hockey injuries. All leagues now require helmets, which must be able to withstand impact from the puck as well as players, boards, and ice. Mouthguards are mandatory in all but international play, and they should be internal and cover all of the teeth of one jaw. A proper mouthguard reduces the frequency of dental injury and may reduce concussion incidence. Full face masks are mandatory in all youth and college leagues and are becoming more popular in professional hockey. USA Hockey recommends hockey equipment certification- (HECC) approved mouthguards, helmets, and facemasks. Many leagues and countries require Kevlar throat protectors. Gloves and elbow, shoulder, shin, and hip pads are all recommended, as are protective cups and tendon pads. Goalkeepers also wear specialized leg guards, a chest protector, a throat protector, a cup, goalie skates, a full face mask, a blocker worn on the stick hand, and a padded trapper.

Knee injuries are the most common lower extremity injuries in hockey. ACL injury is much less common in hockey because the foot may freely slide on the ice. MCL injuries (see Question 63) are approximately 14 times as common due to valgus stress. Thigh contusions (see Question 61), adductor, and groin strain (see Question 56 and 57) are also common in hockey. Groin pain has many possible causes. Prevention of groin strain includes core strengthening and a solid lower extremity stretching program. Ankle injuries (see Question 72) are less common because of the support provided by hockey skates, but they constitute about 10% of injuries requiring more than 28 days of sport abstinence. In contrast to other sports in which lateral ankle sprains are more common, medial ankle sprains are the more common ankle injury in hockey. The common mechanism of an ankle sprain in hockey is eversion, plantar flexion, and internal rotation leading to sprain of the deltoid ligament. Because of this mechanism, a syndesmodic, or high ankle sprain, is also more common, as is proximal fibular fracture. The dorsal foot is also commonly injured in hockey, either by laceration from skates or impingement of tight laces on the dorsum of the foot, which can irritate nerves or tendons. Numbness or burning in the toes or top of the foot should cause you to suspect lace injuries. Lacerations to the foot should be examined by a physician to rule out nerve and tendon injury. Maintaining the tongue of the skate in a neutral position rather than turning it down offers some protection from these injuries.

Injuries to the head, eye, and face (see Questions 21 through 26) are common in hockey. Concussions represent about 7.5% of hockey injuries, and most commonly occur during axial loading when the head strikes another player or the boards. Concussions may also be caused by the puck or ice. Any trauma to the head that results in headache, dizziness, confusion, or nausea should be evaluated by a physician. Face, eye, and dental injuries are also quite common, and may frequently be avoided by wearing the appropriate protective gear. Hockey, in fact, accounts for approximately 40% of all sports-related dental injuries. Studies support that at least half of hockey-related head and face injuries can be prevented by headgear and mouthpieces.

Hockey, in fact, accounts for approximately 40% of all sports-related dental injuries.

Hockey players also commonly injure the neck and back (see Questions 29 through 31 and 51). Because they skate in a forward flexed position, hockey players are prone to muscular and ligamentous back injuries as well as herniated disks. The frequent twisting when skating or striking the puck may also make hockey players more prone to spondylolysis and subsequent spondylolisthesis. A solid core strengthening program may help to reduce back injuries. **Cervical spine** injuries resulting in neck pain should be examined prior to return to play, particularly if there is any involved numbness, weakness, or tingling.

Cervical spine
The neck, consisting of eight vertebrae.

Shoulder injuries are also common in hockey, but may present differently than in other sports. High-velocity collisions, especially with the boards, make shoulder separation or dislocation and clavicle fracture (see Questions 32 through 34) more common in hockey than in most sports.

Hand injuries often occur when gloves are removed for fighting, and gamekeeper's thumb, or ulnar collateral ligament injury (see Question 44), may occur with stick handling if the thumb is hyperabducted. Hockey players may also suffer from pain and numbness of the thumb and dorsal wrist, if the superficial radial nerve is damaged by a stick strike to the wrist. Longer glove cuffs provide some protection from this injury.

Lastly, because of the high forces transferred during hockey collisions, trauma to the chest and abdomen are common. Commotio cordis, or sudden cardiac arrest as discussed in Question 77, has been reported. Automatic electrical defibrillator (AED) use in the setting of commotio cordis may increase survival from this condition to 16%. For this reason, some leagues or team physicians provide AEDs beside the rink.

94. What are the most common volleyball injuries, and how can I prevent them?

Volleyball is a very accessible sport that is enjoyed by men and women of all ages across the United States. It may be played with as few as four persons, on nearly any surface, and requires limited equipment and space.

Because volleyball involves repeated leaping, overhead strikes, and ball-to-hand contact, volleyball injuries tend to fall into specific patterns, including both acute injury and overuse injuries.

Lower extremity injuries include both acute knee and ankle injuries and overuse injuries of the knees and feet. Acute injuries commonly include ankle sprains (see Question 72) and ligamentous or meniscal injury to the knee (see Questions 63, 64, and 67). Overuse injuries commonly include patellar or quadriceps tendonitis (see Question 62), plantar fasciitis (see Question 75), or in rarer cases, stress fractures in the bones of the feet. As with most sports, intensity, duration and frequency of play should be slowly increased.

Appropriate warm-up and stretching prior to exercise is appropriate. Those prone to ankle injuries should wear braces during play, and they should pay attention to appropriate rehabilitation of old injuries. Women especially are prone to ACL injuries and may benefit from an ACL injury prevention program (see Question 64).

The playing surface and equipment play a role both in acute and overuse injuries. Shoes should be appropriate for the foot of the athlete, and should be replaced at regular intervals. The playing surface should be flat, dry, even, and not overly hard. Sand is ideal for avoiding injuries, followed by wood. Concrete is suboptimal.

Shoulder injuries are typically from rotator cuff damage that is sustained as the hand is accelerated from a fully abducted position. These repetitive, high-velocity motions will result in rotator cuff tendonitis and shoulder instability (see Questions 32 and 34). Volleyball players may complain of pain at first only with overhead strikes, which progresses to pain at rest and difficulty lifting the arm or reaching behind the head. Prevention includes rotator cuff strengthening and scapular stabilization programs (see Question 32), as well as discontinuing painful activities, rather than playing through pain. Compared to most athletes, volleyball players are at greater risk of injury to the **suprascapular nerve**, which travels over the shoulder blade to innervate the rotator cuff. Injury to this nerve may easily be confused with severe rotator cuff tendonitis or tear, as it also causes pain and weakness with external rotation and abduction. Your doctor may look for atrophy of the supraspinatus and infraspinatus, confirm your diagnosis with electrical nerve studies (EMG), and/or order an MRI.

Suprascapular nerve

A nerve on the top of the shoulder that is often injured by stretching from a backpack or a direct blow on top of the shoulder as with a lacrosse stick.

The floater serve, in which the player stops the overhead follow-through immediately after striking the ball, is thought to exacerbate this condition.

Frequent jumping and landing in a flexed position also commonly causes back pain in volleyball players. As in most athletes, pain may be from muscular or ligamentous strain, herniated disk, or spondylolysis and spondylolisthesis (see Questions 18, 51, and 54). Like most back pain, a solid core strengthening program can be both preventive and therapeutic. The playing surface also plays a role in back pain.

Hand injuries often occur in volleyball players as a result of misstrikes of the ball. Sprains and strains are most common, followed by contusions, fractures, and dislocations. Gamekeeper's thumb (see Question 44) and finger injuries are common (see Question 45). Wrist injuries occur as acute sprains or strains or in the form of overuse injuries (see Question 41). Medial elbow pain may represent medial epicondylitis, or golfer's elbow (see Question 38). This is commonly exacerbated during overhead serves, because the ball is struck forcefully and the wrist is flexed. Prevention, as with most overuse injuries, involves stretching and strengthening the involved muscle groups. Forearm bands may also be used during play to change the force distribution in the muscle group.

95. What are the most common rowing injuries, and how can I prevent them?

Rowing is generally acknowledged as one of the most strenuous sports and requires both great aerobic capacity and strength. Partly because of the aerobic fitness imparted by rowing, competitive and recreational rowing are rapidly growing in popularity. Competitive rowing takes place in boats that hold one, two, four or eight occupants. It usually has two seasons, a sprint season with sprint races covering distances of 1000–2000 meters, and a fall season with timed head races covering 3 miles. Each rower places his or her feet in fixed shoes, sits on a sliding seat, and employs oars that are fixed in an outrigger. The outrigger can typically be manipulated to alter multiple stroke variables from height and angle to load.

Because rowing is a noncontact sport that requires a highly patterned repetitive rowing motion, nearly all rowing injuries are overuse injuries. The rowing stroke begins with the catch, with the back and legs maximally flexed and arms extended, just as the oars enter the water. From this position, the rower rapidly extends his or her legs and back, and the arms are flexed to the chest, often with the wrists extended. This is termed the drive. The finish occurs as the oar is removed from the water, feathered, or turned parallel to the water, and returned to the catch position.

The drive of the legs and back from a flexed to extended position imparts significant strain on the back and knees. Back injuries resulting from rowing include muscular and ligamentous strain, disk herniation, spondylolysis, and spondylolisthesis (see Questions 18, 51, and 54). As with any sport, rowing mechanics should be carefully examined, and activity should increase in a graduated fashion with regards to distance, intensity, and frequency. Core strengthening may reduce the frequency of back injury. Back problems may also be caused by poor fit of the rower to the seat.

Because rowing maximally loads the knee in its most flexed position, knee injury from rowing most commonly is patellofemoral in nature (see Question 62). Foot positioning within the rowing shell may contribute to the problem and should be examined. Strengthening the vastus medialis and improving hamstring and quadriceps flexibility may help to prevent patellofemoral symptoms. Tendonitis of the knee may also occur, both at the quadriceps and patellar tendons. An appropriate stretching and strengthening program along with a graduated increase in rowing training is also appropriate to prevent these injuries.

Other common pathologies include wrist injuries and nerve compression syndromes. Overuse injury of the wrist and forearm most commonly affects the extensors, which are overtaxed at the end of the drive, and with rapid feathering. To avoid these tendinopathies, modify your rowing technique by loosening your grip on the oar and trying to maintain a neutral wrist position and by avoiding hyperextension during terminal drive and feathering.

Nerve compression syndromes may include individual compression in the nerves supplying the fingers and carpal tunnel syndrome (see Question 43). Compression syndromes in the hand and wrist frequently arise from the same tight grip and repeated hyperextension that cause tendon pathology and may respond to the same preventive measures.

Advanced stress fractures may be detected on plain films (X-rays), but early or subtle fractures may require bone scan for diagnosis.

Lastly, the chronic repeated pull of the serratus anterior on the ribs may cause stress fractures of the ribs, most commonly ribs five through nine in the posterior lateral area. Rib stress fracture may be manifest as chronic chest wall pain, present with activity only at first, but eventually progressing to rest pain. You may have tenderness to palpation over the involved area. Advanced stress fractures may be detected on plain films (X-rays), but early or subtle fractures may require bone scan for diagnosis. Your doctor will recommend appropriate treatment. To avoid stress fractures, increase your activity slowly with regards to frequency, duration, and intensity, and avoid exercising through chest wall pain that is recurrent.

96. What are the most common boxing injuries, and how can I prevent them?

The most common injuries associated with boxing include the following:

- Concussions and other head injuries (see Question 21)
- Facial, jaw, eye, and nose injuries (see Questions 24 through 26)

- Loose, broken, or knocked-out teeth (see Question 28)
- Scrapes, cuts, chafing, and road rash (see Question 13)
- Injuries to the chest, back, and trunk (see Questions 48 through 51)
- Wrist injuries (see Question 41)
- Hand fractures, especially **boxer's fracture**
- Chronic traumatic synovitis
- Elbow injuries (especially ulnar collateral ligament sprain)
- Shoulder injuries (see Questions 32 through 34)
- Overtraining (see Question 15)

Boxer's fracture

Fracture of the metacarpal (knuckle) of the small finger of the hand.

Most injuries encountered in boxing involve blows to the head or face. Concussions, facial lacerations, nose injuries, as well as teeth and jaw injuries, can all be prevented with proper equipment regulations and use. This includes using headgear and mouth guards (mouthpieces) and observing glove size regulations. Chest guards and groin protectors protect against other injuries. Newer boxing gloves and wraps help prevent hand and wrist injuries, although these still remain common during training activities without gloves. Proper punching, blocking, and defensive techniques are important for the boxer to be able to protect himself or herself from injury in the ring.

Additionally, improperly treated acute injuries can lead to long-standing, more difficult to treat, or even permanent problems. For example, swelling and pain are common in the joints of the hand after overdoing it or striking a hard surface with the unprotected fist. This is most common in the knuckles. However, instead of treating the injury with PRICEMM (see Question 10), many athletes tough it out, train through the pain and swelling, and keep pounding away on the injured joints or knuckles. This can lead to a chronic swelling in the joints called chronic traumatic synovitis, which can break down the ligaments that hold the joint together, leading to deformity, chronic pain and swelling, stiffness, and a debilitating loss of the ability to use one's hand. So make sure you take the time out to treat your injuries and seek help from your healthcare professional if you are unsure of how to do so.

Finally, rules and regulations enforced by competition officials are often established in order to protect the athletes and to make the sport as safe as possible. However, they only work if the athletes abide by them, so make sure you follow the rules set by the competition officials.

97. What are the most common karate, kickboxing, kung fu, tae kwon do, wrestling, judo, and aikido injuries, and how can I prevent them?

The most common injuries associated with martial arts and wrestling include:

- Concussions and other head injuries (see Question 21)
- Facial, jaw, eye, and nose injuries (see Questions 24 through 26)
- Ear injuries (especially in wrestling; see Question 27)
- Loose, broken, or knocked-out teeth (see Question 28)
- Neck injuries, including burners or stingers (see Questions 29 through 31)
- Back pain (see Questions 51 through 54)
- Contusions (see Question 61)
- Scrapes, cuts, chafing, and road rash (see Question 13)
- Injuries to the chest, back, and trunk (see Questions 48 through 51)
- Patellofemoral pain syndrome, patellar tendonitis, and quadriceps tendonitis (see Question 62)
- Ankle sprains (see Question 72)
- Achilles tendon problems (see Questions 71 and 74)
- Shoulder injuries (see Questions 32 through 34)
- Elbow injuries (especially ulnar collateral ligament sprain)

- Wrist injuries (see Question 41)
- Hand fractures, especially boxer's fracture
- Finger injuries (see Questions 44 and 45)
- Chronic traumatic synovitis
- Stress fractures (see Question 70)
- Overtraining (see Question 15)

There are several safety measures that can be helpful in preventing martial arts and wrestling injuries and in keeping lost time from training and competition to a minimum. For example, certain techniques or practices are difficult to control at full speed, such as jumping or flying kicks, spinning kicks, axe kicks, certain joint locks. Rules prohibiting or limiting the use of these techniques, as well as adequate protective equipment (especially if these techniques will be allowed in competition) can prevent injuries from these maneuvers. Blows to the head or face place the athlete at higher risk for injury. Concussions, facial lacerations, nose injuries, as well as teeth and jaw injuries can all be prevented with proper equipment regulations and use. Another cause for injuries in martial arts is inadequate training of the athlete, or even a mismatch of skill and fitness between competitors. If a less skilled martial artist is competing against a one who has not been trained to control his or her techniques, there is an increased risk for injury in both participants. Attention paid to teaching martial artists and wrestlers good technique, control, awareness, and strategies to protect themselves will help prevent injuries. Inadequate or improperly fitted or used protective equipment can lead to unsafe situations. Make sure all pads, shields, groin cups, mouthpieces and other equipment are well fitted and in good repair. Depending on the particular sport and rules of the event officials, protective equipment is desirable. This may include head protection, face guards, mouthpieces, eyewear, ear protection, chest and trunk pads, elbow and knee pads, groin cups, shin and forearm pads, fist pads or gloves and instep pads or foam boots. The use of shock-absorbing mats is a must for wrestling and other grappling activities. And always remember to stretch and condition regularly, as well to warm up before participation.

As with boxing injuries (see Question 96), improperly treated acute injuries suffered in the martial arts and wrestling can lead to long-standing, more difficult to treat, or even permanent problems.

Finally, rules and regulations enforced by competition officials are often established in order to protect the athletes, and to make the sports as safe as possible. However, they only work if the athletes abide by them, so make sure you follow the rules set by the competition officials.

98. Can I wrestle with this rash?

Rashes and other skin problems receive a unique amount of attention in wrestling and other grappling sports because of the possibility of infectious causes and the resulting high risk of spreading the infection. In addition to causing unnecessary lost competition time for other athletes, the athlete with a rash can also develop a worsening of the rash or even a second infection on top of the first one if appropriate measures are not taken. Infection may spread through skin contact, from both another person and from the mat. Most organized venues for wrestling or other grappling events will have well established rules for who can and who cannot participate with a rash. These regulations are often patterned after those used by the NCAA for collegiate level wrestling. In general, the decision is ultimately up to the covering healthcare provider or athletic trainer. See your healthcare provider if you have a rash and still want to participate in an event such as wrestling. The first thing the healthcare professional will do is ask you details about your rash, perform an examination, perhaps order tests on samples of your skin, and decide whether or not your rash is infectious. If it is not, then you will probably be allowed to return to training and competition with appropriate treatment and protection of the affected skin. However, if the cause is

Infection may spread through skin contact, from both another person and from the mat.

determined to be infectious, the NCAA has the following specific rules as to how long you need to be treated before returning to participation:

- Bacterial infections—like impetigo or cellulites—must be treated with an antibiotic medication for at least 72 hours, with no new skin or wet lesions for 48 hours.
- Fungal infections on the skin must be treated with a topical antifungal medication for at least 72 hours, with no new skin lesions for 48 hours. Infections in the scalp must be treated with an oral antifungal medication for 2 weeks.
- Viral infections—like herpes, molluscum contagiosum, or warts—need to be treated with an antiviral medication for at least 120 hours, with no new skin lesions for 72 hours. Molluscum contagiosum lesions must be removed by a healthcare provider prior to competition.
- Infections from mites and scabies must be completely treated and resolved.

In general, in order for the athlete to return to wrestling, all skin lesions need to be dry with no oozing or discharge. When the athlete returns to play, he or she must keep the remaining lesions covered and protected while participating, with apparel, bandages, or tape. When covering fungal rashes before competition, the skin lesions should be washed with an antifungal shampoo, dressed with a topical antifungal medication, and finally protected and secured with gauze and tape.

The best way to prevent skin infections in wrestling and other grappling sports is good personal hygiene, using properly disinfected wrestling mats and equipment, prompt recognition and treatment of skin problems, and abiding by the rules set by your sport's organizational body.

99. What are the most common cheerleading injuries, and how can I prevent them?

Current-day cheerleading is a highly demanding activity that not only supports the teams from the sideline, but involves competition at a very high level among themselves year round. Gone are the days of simple pom-poms and organizing cheers. Modern-day cheerleading is more like high-level gymnastics in addition to the traditional cheers.

With its skyrocketing participation and competition to push the envelope of safety, cheerleading is considered by many to be one of the most dangerous sports. Cheerleading injuries have increased dramatically in recent years and were estimated to account for 25,000 hospital visits in 2001. In an injury survey in 1997 looking at severe and fatal injuries from 1982 to 1997, cheerleading ranked No. 1 for both the high school and college level. A major factor in this increase is the high-level gymnastic routines, use of mini trampolines, and pyramid building.

Common cheerleading-related injuries include ankle sprains (see Question72), back and neck injuries (see Questions 18, 30, and 51), head injuries including concussion (see Question 21), knee injuries (see Questions 62 through 65 and 67), and elbow injuries. Injury patterns are related to the specific skills that include dancing, gymnastic and partner stunts. The most dangerous are the gymnastic and partner stunts that include lifts, pyramid building, and tossing. Discussion of the management of these various injuries has been discussed previously in this book. The development of these injuries will depend on the stunts attempted and the cheerleader's position as a base or top of the pyramid or being tossed in certain stunts. Other contributing factors include inadequate conditioning, poor supervision, noncushioned ground surfaces, poor quality shoes and nutrition, and lack of experience.

Recommendations to make cheerleading safer include:

1. *Supervision*—Coaches should be trained and certified; they should read and adhere to the American Association of Cheerleading Coaches and Advisors safety guidelines for the appropriate competition level. The National Federation of State High School Associations publishes the *Spirit Rule Book,* a safety resource for coaches. Practice and performance should be done only under the coaches' supervision. Coaches should ensure proper technique as well as spotters for higher risk moves and mounting; they should teach gradual progression of difficult skills; and they must ensure there is a good emergency plan for injuries.
2. *Equipment*—Cheerleaders should practice on mats or pads and wear proper shoes.
3. *General health*—Cheerleaders and coaches should recognize eating disorders and the female athlete triad (see Question 1). Injuries should be identified, treated, and properly rehabilitated. Cheerleaders are athletes and they should have a preseason evaluation. In a 1997 article in *Phys Sportsmed*, Hutchinson asserted that cheerleaders should progress through flexibility and strengthening drills. All cheerleaders should specifically work on core strengthening, and those athletes who will be on the base of pyramids should work on rotator cuff strengthening.

100. Where or how can I get more information?

The following Web sites provide additional information.

University of Michigan—Sports Medicine Health Topics: This site includes an online version of the *Sports Medicine Advisor*, a book with general information on various sports medicine topics, injuries, and rehabilitation.

http://www.med.umich.edu/1libr/sma/sma_index.htm

The Athletic Advisor: This site has a good amount of general information on athletic training and injury treatment and prevention. This site was originally developed by an athletic trainer for use by high schools without the benefit of an athletic trainer or sports medicine physician.

http://www.athleticadvisor.com/

About.com—Sports Medicine and Health: This site includes a collection of short articles providing general information on various sports medicine topics, injuries, rehabilitation, etc.

http://sportsmedicine.about.com/

The Stretching Institute: This is the Web site for a company that produces several educational resources on sports medicine-related topics. This site includes access to articles on stretching, injury prevention, and rehabilitation of sports-related injuries.

http://www.thestretchinghandbook.com/

FootSmart: This is a great Web site belonging to an Internet vendor that specializes in products related to foot and lower extremity health, including braces, orthotic inserts, heel cups, and other products. Athletes can search the site by condition or symptom.

http://www.footsmart.com/Page.aspx?pageId=12

American Medical Society for Sports Medicine (AMSSM): This is the home page for the AMSSM, a national organization of sports medicine experts in the full spectrum of caring for athletes. The site includes a searchable list of physicians who either specialize in or have a strong interest in caring for athletes and the active individual.

http://www.amssm.org/

Exercises

Figure 1: Neck Exercises

If any of these exercises significantly worsen your pain, stop doing them and contact you healthcare provider.

Stretching and Range of Motion

1. NECK ROTATION STRETCH: Turn your head slowly to the left, moving it gently to the point of pain, and holding it there for about 3 seconds. Then, move it back to a straight-forward position, relax, and take a deep breath. Next, repeat the procedure toward the right, and returning to the straight-forward position, relax and breathe. This is one repetition. Do at least two sets of ten repetitions a day.

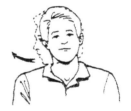

2. NECK SIDE-BENDING STRETCH: Tilt your head slowly towards the left shoulder, moving it gently to the point of pain and making sure you do not turn your head while you do so. Hold that position for about 3 seconds. Then, move your head back to a straight-forward position, relax, and take a deep breath. Next, repeat the procedure towards the right, and returning to the straight-forward position, relax and breathe. This is one repetition. Do at least two sets of ten repetitions a day.

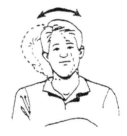

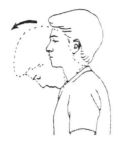

3. NECK FLEXION STRETCH: Bend your head slowly forward, bringing your chin toward your chest, moving it gently to the point of pain, and holding it there for about 5 seconds. Then, move your head back to a straight-forward position, relax, and take a deep breath. This is one repetition. Do at least two sets of ten repetitions a day.

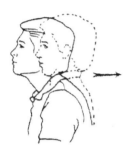

4. NECK EXTENSION STRETCH: Tilt your head slowly back, pointing your chin towards the sky, moving it gently to the point of pain, and holding it there for about 5 seconds. Then, move your head back to a straight-forward position, relax, and take a deep breath. This is one repetition. Do at least two sets of ten repetitions a day.

5. CHIN TUCKS: Gently push your head straight back, tucking your chin in as if to make a double chin. **Do not look up or down with your face.** Hold that position for about 5 seconds. Then, move your head back to a neutral position, relax, and take a deep breath. This is one repetition. Do at least two sets of five repetitions a day.

6. TRAPEZIUS STRETCH: With your right arm behind your lower back, look toward the affected side and with the opposite hand pull your head toward the thigh of the same leg as the hand on the head. Hold this gentle stretch for about 30 seconds. Then, move your head back to a neutral position, relax, and take a deep breath. Repeat the process for the other side. This is one repetition. Do at least two sets of three repetitions a day.

Strengthening

1. NECK ISOMETRIC FLEXION: Place the palm of your hand against your forehead, gently push your forehead into your hand, holding for about 5 seconds. Then, move your head back to a neutral position, relax, and take a deep breath. This is one repetition. Do at least three sets of five repetitions a day.

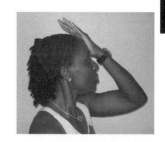

2. NECK ISOMETRIC EXTENSION: Clasp your hands and fingers together behind your head, gently press the back of your head into your hands, holding for about 5 seconds. Then, move your head back to a neutral position, relax, and take a deep breath. This is one repetition. Do at least three sets of five repetitions a day.

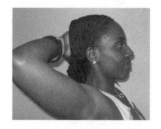

3. NECK ISOMETRIC SIDE-BENDING: Place the palm of your hand against the side of your head and gently push your head into your hand, holding for about 5 seconds. Then, move your head back to a neutral position, relax, and take a deep breath. This is one repetition. Do at least three sets of five repetitions a day.

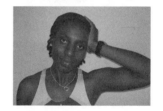

Figure 2: Shoulder–Strengthening Exercises

Perform all exercises with a 2-4 lb weight. Hold each position for 5 seconds and perform three sets of ten repetitions.

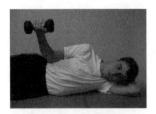

EXTERNAL ROTATION: With the weight on the floor and elbow tight to the side lift the weight until it is just above horizontal and hold.

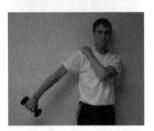

ABDUCTION: Starting with the arm hanging at your side, raise the arm to 30-45 degrees and hold. Your thumb should be pointed down. Emphasize not elevating the shoulder. This can be aided by placing the opposite hand on the shoulder to keep it down while performing the repetitions.

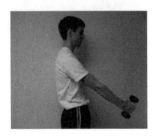

FORWARD ELEVATION: Starting with the arm hanging at your side raise the arm forward to 30-45 degrees with the thumb pointing up and hold.

Figure 3: Scapular Exercises

Perform these exercises slowly, smoothly, and with control. There should be no jerky movements. If any of the exercises cause pain, discontinue them immediately. When adding weights, start with just a little bit of weight (a small soup can works nicely). If the exercises become too difficult to do with weights, decrease or remove the weights.

STABILIZATION IN PRONE: While lying facedown with elbows straight and arms out-stretched at the sides, raise both arms off the floor and hold for 2 seconds, and then relax. This is one repetition. Start with no weights; once the exercise becomes easier to do, you may add 1-2 lbs to each hand. Perform two to three sets of ten to fifteen repetitions once a day.

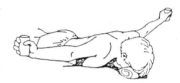

PRONE OR SEATED RETRACTION: While lying facedown and keeping arms out from the sides and elbows bent, pinch or squeeze the shoulder blades together. Hold for 2 seconds, and then relax. This is one repetition. Perform two to three sets of ten to fifteen repetitions once a day.

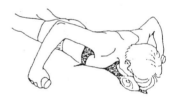

(You may also do this from a sitting position)

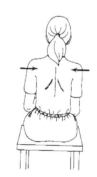

Figure 4: Shoulder Range of Motion After Injury

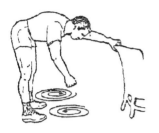

PENDULUM EXERCISES: While resting the unaffected arm on a chair or table, lean forward and let the injured arm hang down. Work the arm in slowly enlarging circles as pain will allow. Perform 2–3 minutes of rotation in a clockwise and counterclockwise direction twice daily for the first few days after injury.

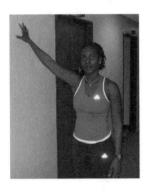

WALL CLIMBS: Stand about three fourths of an arm's length from a wall with the affected arm closest to the wall. Using the fingers of the hand like a "spider," climb up the wall to stretch the joint capsule. When you get to the maximum point you can take based on pain, hold that position for 10 seconds. If you wish, you can even attempt to lift the hand off the wall surface for 5 seconds to activate the rotator cuff muscles. Repeat five times and perform three sets per day.

Figure 5: Shoulder Reduction

SELF-REDUCTION: Fold your arms in front of your bent knee on the same side as the dislocated shoulder. Clasp your hands tightly, but relax your arms and shoulder muscles. Slowly lean back while continuing to relax. The shoulder will make a clunk sound when it reduces.

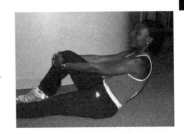

TWO-PERSON REDUCTION: Have the injured individual lie on his or her back with the affected arm out toward the assistant. The assistant places the arch of his or her foot high into the armpit of the injured individual and clasps the forearm. While keeping his or her knees and elbows straight, the assistant leans back, slowly placing a firm, smooth traction on the arm. The injured individual relaxes his or her arm and shoulder muscles as much as possible. The shoulder should make a clunk sound when it reduces and the pain will be significantly reduced.

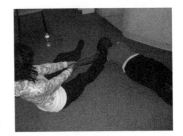

When the shoulder is reduced (when it is back in place), place the arm in a sling and seek medical attention.

Figure 6: Shoulder–Stretching Exercises

These stretches should be performed after warming up the affected shoulder by applying a warm, moist compress for 10 minutes. These exercises should be mildly uncomfortable but not overly painful.

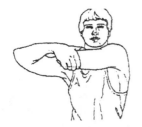

POSTERIOR CAPSULE STRETCH: Grasp the elbow with the opposite hand and pull the arm across the body until you feel a stretching sensation in the back of the shoulder. Hold position for 20 seconds and then release. Repeat for a total of five repetitions.

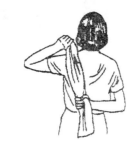

TOWEL STRETCH: Grasp both ends of a rolled towel with the affected arm down. With the upper hand, pull the lower hand up behind the back. Stretch and hold for 15–20 seconds, and then release. Do five repetitions.

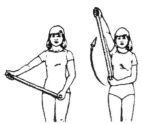

CANE RANGE OF MOTION: Grasp both ends of a cane or 3-foot broom handle. The affected arm is the upper arm. Utilizing pressure from the good arm, push the range of motion or the affected arm. Push up as far as you can go and hold for 15–20 seconds and release. Do five repetitions.

Figure 7: Tennis Elbow Exercises

EXTENSOR STRETCH: With the elbow straight, grasp the fingers and flex the wrist to stretch the muscles of the outside part of the elbow. Hold for 20 seconds and repeat five times.

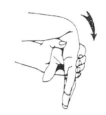

WRIST EXTENSOR STRENGTHENING: Using a 3–4 lb weight and with the palm down, slowly raise the weight. Hold in the up position for 5 seconds. Then slowly lower the weight. Do ten repetitions and three sets per day.

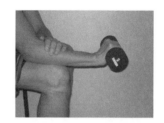

SUPINATOR STRENGTHENING: Hold a hammer near the base of the handle with the palm down and the hammer horizontal. Slowly raise the hammer to the vertical position. Then lower it back to the starting position. Do ten repetitions and three sets per day.

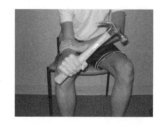

FRICTION MASSAGE: Heat the elbow up with a warm, moist towel for 10 minutes. Identify the area of maximal tenderness in the outside of the elbow and place the thumb of the opposite hand over this area and deeply massage back and forth across the tendon for 3–5 minutes. Perform this massage every 3–4 days. You may ice the elbow for pain produced by this deep–tissue massage.

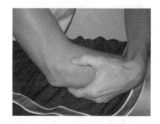

Figure 8: Golfer's Elbow Exercises

Stretching

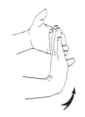

ELBOW FLEXOR STRETCH: With the elbow straight, pull the wrist back to stretch the muscle group on the inside part of the forearm. Hold for 20 seconds and repeat five times.

STRENGTHENING: Hold each following position for 5 seconds and lower slowly to get a negative resistance workout. Perform three sets of ten repetitions.

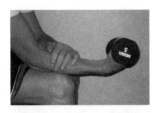

WRIST FLEXOR STRENGTHENING: Use a 2–4 lb weight for strengthening. Rest your forearm on your leg and stabilize it with the opposite hand. Curl the wrist to elevate the weight.

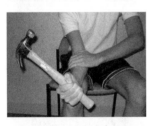

PRONATOR STRENGTHENING: Hold a hammer close to the end of the handle with the palm up and the hammer horizontal. Slowly rotate the hammer 90 degrees until it is straight up. Then slowly return to the starting position.

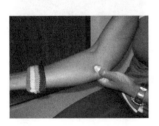

FRICTION MASSAGE: Heat the elbow up with a warm, moist towel for 10 minutes. Identify the area of maximal tenderness on the inside of the elbow and place the thumb of the opposite hand over this area and deeply massage back and forth across the tendon for 3–5 minutes. Perform this massage every 3–4 days. You may ice the elbow for pain produced by this deep-tissue massage.

Figure 9: Acute Back Pain Exercises

Prior to the performance of these exercises, apply heat to your back in the form of a warm, moist towel for 10 minutes. If you have severe spasms, application of ice prior to these stretches may relieve your spasm.

Knee–Chest Stretching

SINGLE LEG: While lying on your back, pull one leg to your chest while the opposite leg is straight. Hold for 20 seconds. Repeat five times.

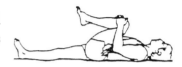

DOUBLE LEG: While lying on your back, pull both legs to your chest and hold for 20 seconds. Repeat five times.

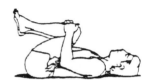

CATBACK: While on all fours, arch your back with your head down and tighten your abdominal and buttock muscles. Hold for 20 seconds and repeat five times.

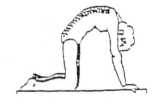

PRESS-UP EXTENSION: Lie on your stomach in push-up position. Slowly raise your body while keeping your hips on the floor. Relax your buttocks. Hold for 20 seconds and repeat five times.

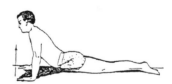

Figure 10: Core Flexibility Exercises

All these stretches should be performed after warming up and should be held for 15 seconds and repeated five times for 1–2 sessions per day

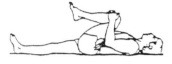

ACTIVE HAMSTRING STRETCH: Lie on your back and bring the thigh up to a vertical position, holding it with your hands. Slowly straighten the knee by contracting the quads and feel the stretch in the back of the thigh.

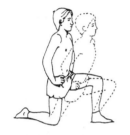

HIP FLEXOR STRETCH: Tighten your abdominal muscles and hold yourself erect, then slowly step forward. Feel the stretching in the front of your hip and thigh.

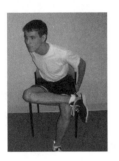

PIRIFORMIS (SEATED): Sit in a chair and cross your legs. Rotate your trunk to center on the thigh of the side you want to stretch. While keeping your head up and back straight or arched slightly, lean toward the thigh. You should feel the stretch deep in your buttocks.

Figure 11: Core Strengthening Exercises

Perform all these exercises after warming up and stretching. Hold each position for 10 seconds and initially perform five repetitions, but plan to increase to ten repetitions per day as you get stronger.

PELVIC TILT: While lying on your back, tighten your lower abdominal muscles to rock your pelvis forward or flatten your back against the floor.

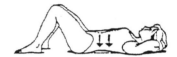

CRUNCH: While lying on your back, cross your arms loosely and tuck your chin down. Tighten the abdominal muscles and curl up until your shoulder blades come off the floor.

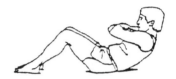

BRIDGE: While lying on your back, without arching your lower back, raise hips upward, keeping a straight line from your knees to your shoulders.

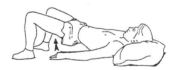

QUADRUPED: While on all fours, lift one arm and the opposite leg, and then put them down. Repeat with the opposite arm and leg. Maintain a neutral tilt of your pelvis.

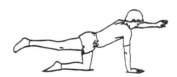

Figure 12: Groin Strain Exercises

After resting for about 2–3 days after your injury, try these stretches as soon as you can tolerate
them.

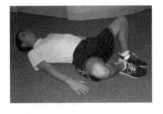

1. HIP ADDUCTOR STRETCH: Lying on
your back with your knees bent and feet flat on
the floor, gently spread your knees apart, until you
feel the stretch inside your hips. Gently take the
stretch barely to the point of pain, holding it there
for about 30 seconds. Then, move your knees and
hips back to the starting position, relax, and take a
deep breath. This is one repetition. Do at least two
sets of three repetitions a day.

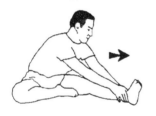

2. SITTING HAMSTRING STRETCH: Sit
with your knee kept straight and lean forward,
reaching for your foot and feeling the stretch in
the back of your thigh. You may feel some discomfort, but there should be no sharp pains. Hold this
position for 15–20 seconds. Then, slowly relax and
return to the starting position. This is one repetition. Do at least two sets of five repetitions on each
leg, each day.

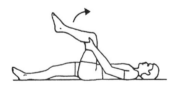

3. ACTIVE HAMSTRING STRETCH: Lie
on your back and bring your thigh up to a vertical position, holding it with your hands. Slowly
straighten the knee by contracting the quads and
feel the stretch in the back of the thigh. Hold for
15–20 seconds and do five repetitions two times
a day.

4. STRAIGHT LEG RAISE: Lying on your back with your hips and one knee bent and the other straight, contract the muscles in the front of the thigh you are planning to strengthen, lifting the heel about 8 inches off the floor. Hold this position for 15–30 seconds, keeping the thigh muscles tight. Then, slowly relax and lower the leg back to the floor. Repeat on the other side. This is one repetition. Do at least three sets of ten repetitions a day.

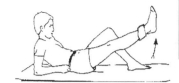

5. SIDE-LYING LEG RAISE: Lying on the side you want to exercise (bottom), bend the other (top) knee and place the corresponding foot in front of the leg you are going to strengthen. Keep the bottom leg straight. Contract the muscles on the inside of the bottom thigh, raising the bottom leg off the floor, as far as you can go without pain. Hold this position for 5–10 seconds, keeping the thigh muscles tight. Then, slowly relax and lower the leg back to the floor. This is one repetition. Do at least three sets of ten repetitions on each leg, each day.

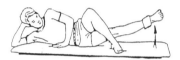

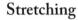

Figure 13: Snapping Hip Exercises

Stretching

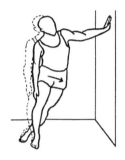

1. SIDE-LEANING ILIOTIBIAL BAND STRETCH: Standing with the side you are planning to stretch near a wall, cross your uninjured leg in front of the leg you are planning to stretch, distributing your weight evenly between the two feet. Using the hand closest to the wall for support, lean your hips into the wall, feeling a stretch on the side of your hip. Hold this position for 15–30 seconds. Then, slowly relax and return to the starting position. This is one repetition. Do at least two sets of three repetitions on each leg, each day.

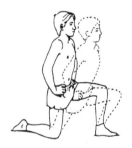

2. HIP FLEXOR STRETCH: Keeping the knee and foot of the hip you are planning to stretch on the floor, move the other leg forward and place its foot flat on the floor. From this position, lean further, leaning forward at the hips, pressing both hips towards the floor. You should feel a stretch in the front of your hip. Hold this position for 15–30 seconds. Then, slowly relax and return to the starting position. This is one repetition. Do at least two sets of three repetitions on each leg, each day.

Strengthening

1. HIP ABDUCTOR STRENGTHENING: Lie on your side with the affected hip up. Keeping the leg straight, raise it about 12–18 inches or 30 degrees from horizontal. Hold for 5 seconds and then slowly lower. Perform three sets of ten repetitions. When this becomes easy, add a 1-lb ankle weight for more resistance.

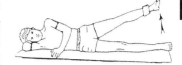

2. HIP FLEXIONS STRENGTHENING: Lie on your back with the affected leg out straight and the other knee bent. Raise the leg at the hip about 12 inches and hold for 5 seconds. Lower the leg slowly to the floor. Perform three sets of ten repetitions. When this becomes easy, add a 1-lb ankle weight for more resistance.

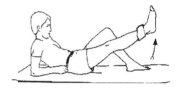

Figure 14: Quad Exercises

Phase 1 uses stretching to address initial pain and swelling. Apply the principles of PRICEMM (questions 10 and 11), and consider a 6-inch compression wrap or a hamstring sleeve that can be purchased online. Once you have no pain walking or climbing up and down stairs, you may begin the phase 2 strengthening exercises, but do not forget to continue the phase 1 stretching exercises as well.

Phase 1—Stretching

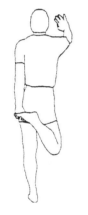

QUADRICEPS STRETCH: Standing in front of a wall, grasp the ankle of the side you are planning to stretch with the hand of the opposite side, and pull the heel towards your buttocks, bending at the knee, and keeping both knees as close together as possible. You may use the opposite hand to brace yourself on the wall for balance. Keep your back straight, without arching backwards or twisting to the side. Hold this position for 15–30 seconds. Then, slowly relax and return to the starting position. This is one repetition. Do at least two sets of three repetitions on each leg, each day.

Phase 2—Strengthening

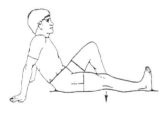

1. QUADRICEPS ISOMETRIC STRENGTHENING: Sit on the floor with the leg you are planning to strengthen straight, and the other knee bent. Contract the muscles in the front of your exercising thigh, pressing the back of the knee into the floor, and hold this position for 10–15 seconds. Then, slowly relax. This is one repetition. Do at least three sets of ten repetitions on each leg, each day.

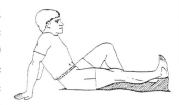

2. STRAIGHT LEG RAISE: Leaning back on your hands while sitting on the ground with the affected knee straight and the other bent at 90 degrees, contract the muscles in the front of the thigh you are planning to strengthen, lifting the heel about 8 inches off the floor. Hold this position for 15–30 seconds, keeping the thigh muscles tight. Then, slowly relax and lower the leg back to the floor. Repeat on the other side. This is one repetition. Do at least three sets of ten repetitions per day.

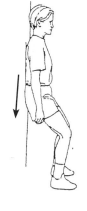

3. QUADRICEPS WALL SLIDE: Stand with the back of your head, shoulders, back, and hips against a wall. Place your feet one shoulder's width apart and about 1 foot away from the wall. As a guide, you may also place a rolled-up pillow or a soccer ball between your knees. Keeping your head against the wall, but your neck and shoulders relaxed, slowly slide your back and hips down to-wards the floor. Tighten the muscles in the front of your thigh and those in your buttocks. Continue to lower your body until your thighs are parallel to the floor. Hold this position for 10–30 seconds. Then, slowly raise your body back up to the start-ing position, keeping your thighs and buttocks tight the whole way. Finally, relax and take a deep breath. This is one repetition. Do three sets of ten repetitions a day.

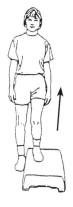

4. STEPS: Stand in front of a set of stairs, and slowly step up onto the first step first with the leg you plan to exercise. Once both feet are on the step, slowly step back down, keeping your weight on the exercising foot, on the first step. Relax and take a deep breath. This is one repetition. Do three sets of ten repetitions, on each leg, a day.

Figure 15: Hamstring Exercises

Phase 1, stretching, is to address initial pain and swelling. Apply the principles of PRICEMM (questions 10 and 11) and consider a 6-inch compression wrap or a hamstring sleeve that can be purchased online. Once you have no pain walking or climbing up and down stairs, you may begin the phase 2 strengthening exercises, but do not forget to continue the phase 1 stretching exercises as well.

Phase 1—Stretching

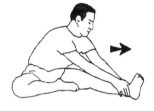

1. SITTING HAMSTRING STRETCH: While sitting with one knee kept straight and one foot touching the opposite thigh, lean forward reaching for your outstretched foot, feeling the stretch in the back of the thigh. You may feel some discomfort, but there should be no sharp pains. Hold this position for 15–20 seconds. Then, slowly relax and return to the starting position. This is one repetition. Do at least two sets of five repetitions on each leg, each day.

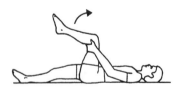

2. ACTIVE HAMSTRING STRETCH: Lie on your back and bring the thigh up to a vertical position, holding it with your hands. Slowly straighten the knee by contracting the thigh muscles and feel the stretch in the back of the thigh. Hold for 15–20 seconds and do five repetitions two times a day.

Phase 2—Strengthening

1. PRONE KNEE BENDS: Lying face down with both legs straight, slowly bend the knee you are planning to exercise and bring the heel towards your buttocks. Hold this position for 5–10 seconds. Then, slowly return your leg to the starting position, relax, and take a deep breath. This is one repetition. Do three sets of ten repetitions, on both legs, each day. You may add ankle weights to make this exercise more challenging.

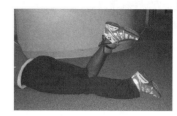

2. PRONE HIP EXTENSIONS: Lying face down with both legs straight, slowly tighten the muscles of the buttock you are planning to exercise, keep your knee straight, and lift that leg about 8 inches off the floor. Hold this position for 5–10 seconds. Then, slowly return your leg to the starting position, relax, and take a deep breath. This is one repetition. Do three sets of ten repetitions, on both legs, each day. You may add ankle weights to make this exercise more challenging.

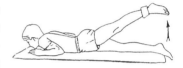

3. HEEL SLIDE: sit on the floor with both legs straight. Slowly slide the heel of the leg you are planning to exercise towards your buttock, pulling the knee towards your chest. Hold this position for a few seconds. Then, slowly relax and return to the starting position. This is one repetition. Do at least three sets of ten repetitions on each leg, each day.

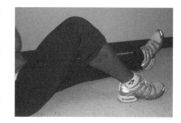

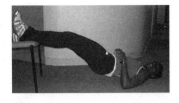

4. CHAIR LIFTS: Lying on your back with both heels on top of a chair, stool, or lowered table, slowly tighten the muscles in the back of your thighs and buttocks, and raise both hips off of the floor. Hold this position for 2–5 seconds. Then, slowly return your hips to the starting position, keeping your muscles tight. Relax and take a deep breath. This is one repetition. Do three sets of fifteen to twenty repetitions a day.

Figure 16: Patellofemoral Exercises

For patellofemoral pain syndrome (PFPS), the hamstring stretches, straight leg raise, quadriceps wall slide, steps, iliotibial band stretches, and Muncie modified straight-leg raises are very helpful.

Stretching

1. SITTING HAMSTRING STRETCH: While sitting with one knee kept straight and one foot touching the opposite thigh, lean forward, reaching for your foot, feeling the stretch in the back of the thigh. You may feel some discomfort, but there should be no sharp pains. Hold this position for 15–20 seconds. Then, slowly relax and return to the starting position. This is one repetition. Do at least two sets of five repetitions on each leg, each day.

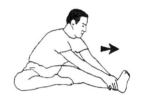

2. ACTIVE HAMSTRING STRETCH: Lie on your back and bring the thigh up to a vertical position, holding it with your hands. Slowly straighten the knee by contracting the thigh muscles and feel the stretch in the back of the thigh. Hold for 15–20 seconds and repeat five repetitions two times a day.

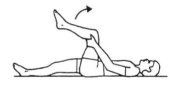

3. SIDE-LEANING ILIOTIBIAL BAND STRETCH: Standing with the side you are planning to stretch near a wall, cross your uninjured leg in front of the leg you are planning to stretch, distributing your weight evenly between the two feet. Using the hand closest to the wall for support, lean your hips into the wall, feeling a stretch on the side of your hip. Hold this position for 15–30

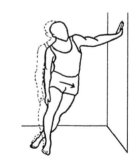

seconds. Then, slowly relax and return to the starting position. This is one repetition. Do at least two sets of three repetitions on each leg, each day.

Strengthening

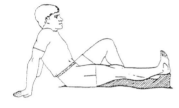

1.. STRAIGHT LEG RAISE: Sit on the floor with the knee you are planning to strengthen straight and the other bent; contract the muscles in the front of the thigh you are planning to strengthen, lifting the heel about 8 inches off the floor. Hold this position for 15–30 seconds, keeping the thigh muscles tight. Then, slowly relax and lower the leg back to the floor. Repeat on the other side. This is one repetition. Do at least three sets of ten repetitions a day.

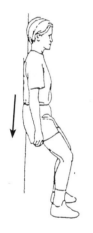

2. QUADRICEPS WALL SLIDE: Stand with the back of your head, shoulders, back, and hips against a wall. Place your feet one shoulder's width apart and about 1 foot away from the wall. As a guide, you may also place a rolled-up pillow or a soccer ball between your knees. Keeping your head against the wall, but your neck and shoulders relaxed, slowly slide your back and hips down towards the floor. Tighten the muscles in the front of your thigh and those in your buttocks. Continue to lower your body until your thighs are parallel to the floor. Hold this position for 10–30 seconds. Then, slowly raise your body back up to the starting position, keeping your thighs and buttocks tight the whole way. Finally, relax and take a deep breath. This is one repetition. Do three sets of ten repetitions per day.

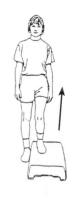

3 STEPS: Stand in front of a set of stairs, and slowly step up onto the first step first with the leg you plan to exercise, and then with the other leg. Once both feet are on the step, slowly step back down, keeping your weight on the exercising foot, on the first step. Relax and take a deep breath. This is one repetition. Do three sets of ten repetitions, on each leg, each day.

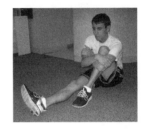

4 MODIFIED STRAIGHT-LEG RAISES (MUNCIE METHOD): Sit on the floor with the knee you are planning to exercise straightened. Bend the nonexercising knee so that the foot is flat on the floor and about even with the exercising knee. Give the bent knee a hug, lean forward, and turn the exercising leg out slightly so that your big toe points to the 2 o'clock position (10 o'clock if it's your left leg). Now, raise the exercising leg slowly about 1 inch off the ground by tightening the muscles in the front of your thigh, keeping the knee straight. Hold this position for 5 seconds. Then, slowly return your legs to the starting position, relax, and take a deep breath. This is one repetition. Do twenty good repetitions each day. Note that the closer your chest is to the thigh, the harder the exercise.

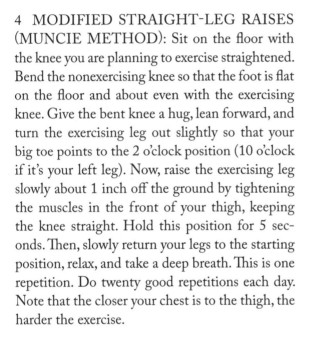

Figure 17: Exercises for Shin Splints

Stretching

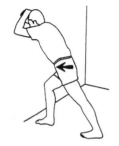

1. STANDING GASTROCNEMIUS CALF STRETCH: Standing in front of a wall place both hands on the wall, and step back with the leg you are planning to stretch, keeping the other, supporting leg forward and bent at the knee. Turn the foot of your stretching leg inward (so that your toes are pointing at the wall). Keep the stretching leg's heel on the floor. Now, slowly lean forward and feel the gentle stretch in the back of your calf. Hold the stretch for 15–30 seconds. Then relax and take a deep breath. This is one repetition. Do several sets of three repetitions for each leg, each day.

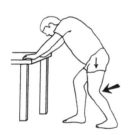

2. STANDING SOLEUS STRETCH: This exercise is performed the same way as the standing calf stretch in step 1, except you keep the stretching leg's knee slightly bent. You will feel the stretch in a different area in the back of your calf. Once again, it is important to keep the stretching leg's heel to the floor and the foot turned slightly inward.

Strengthening

1. INVERSION STRENGTHENING: While lying on your back, press inward with the affected foot against the other foot, a wall or a door jamb. Hold for 10 seconds. Perform three sets of ten-repetitions.

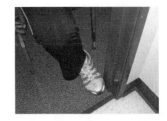

2. DORSIFLEXION STRENGTHENING: While lying on your back with a pillow on the affected foot, resist the upward motion of the foot of the affected leg with the other foot. Attempt to lift the foot up for 10 seconds. Perform three sets of ten repetitions.

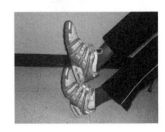

Figure 18: Achilles Tendonitis Exercises

Stretching

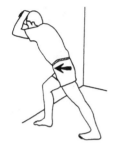

1. STANDING GASTROCNEMIUS (CALF) STRETCH: Standing in front of a wall, place both hands on the wall and step back with the leg you are planning to stretch, keeping the other, supporting leg forward and bent at the knee. Turn the foot of your stretching leg inward (so that your toes are pointing at the wall). Keep the stretching leg's heel on the floor. Now, slowly lean forward and feel the gentle stretch in the back of your calf. Hold the stretch for 15–30 seconds. Then relax and take a deep breath. This is one repetition. Do several sets of three repetitions for each leg, each day.

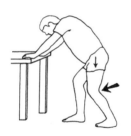

2. STANDING SOLEUS STRETCH: This exercise is performed the same way as the standing calf stretch in step 1, except you keep the stretching leg's knee slightly bent. You will feel the stretch in a different area in the back of your calf. Once again, it is important to keep the stretching leg's heel to the floor and your foot turned slightly inward.

Strengthening

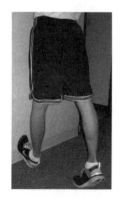

1. HEEL RAISE: While standing behind a chair, table, or in front of a wall for support, slowly contract the muscles in your calves and go up on your toes, raising your heels off the ground as far as you can. Hold this position for 5–10 seconds. Then slowly lower your heels back to the starting position, relax, and take a deep breath. This is one repetition. Do three sets of ten repetitions a day. If this exercise becomes too easy, you can do the exercise with the balls of your feet on a bottom

step and your heels off of the step. You may also perform the exercise on one leg at a time, to make the exercise more challenging.

2. SINGLE-LEG BALANCE: Stand and try to balance on the exercising leg without any support. Hold this position for 30 seconds, then relax and take a deep breath. This is one repetition. Do two sets of three repetitions for each leg, each day. Do this exercise with your eyes open at first. As it gets easier, you may then try the exercise with your eyes closed. Finally, for more of a challenge, try doing the exercise while standing on a folded towel.

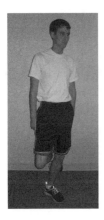 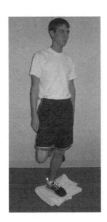

3. HOPPING / JUMPING: Once you can do exercises 1 and 2 without much of a problem, try hopping on one leg across the room and back. Then repeat the exercise using the other leg. This is one repetition. Do two sets of three repetitions for each leg, each day. Once that gets easier, do the exercise while jumping as high as you can each time, as opposed to just hopping. Make sure that you land softly, bending at both the ankle and the knee. Avoid landing hard on your feet and heels.

Figure 19: Ankle Rehabilitation

The rehabilitation of ankle sprains is divided into five phases.

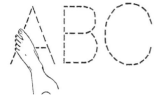

Phase 1 ankle rehabilitation consists of PRICEMM (see questions 10 and 11) and early motion of the ankle: write the capital letters of the alphabet with your big toe by moving the ankle. Only move to the point of a good stretch; some discomfort is normal, but you should not feel sharp pain. Phase 1 rehabilitation usually lasts 3–7 days and the goals are pain management, reduction of swelling and some return of motion.

Phases 2 and 3 ankle rehabilitation consists of more range-of-motion exercises, as well as some strengthening and balance training exercises. When your ankle swelling has improved, and you can stand and walk without too much pain, it is time move into phase 2 rehabilitation. Start with the phase 1 stretching exercises, and then move into the strengthening and balance training exercises as you continue to improve (usually after 1–3 weeks). Ultimately, try to get to the point of doing all the phase 2 and 3 exercises, but if a new exercise causes pain, stop the exercise and try again after a few days. For ankle sprains, you should do the exercises used for calf (gastrocnemius and soleus) stretching and strengthening in addition to the ankle-specific exercises that follow. See Figure 17 for more information on calf strains.

1. ANKLE RANGE OF MOTION: While sitting on the floor or lying on your back with your

legs straight in front of you, slowly move your ankle, pointing your toes towards your head, away from your head, towards the other foot, away from the other foot, and around in circles. Keep all the motion in the ankle, while keeping the leg and knee still. Initially, move gently, but as your symptoms improve, make the movements more firm. Repeat the exercise ten times in each direction. Do this at least twice a day.

2. ISOMETRIC STRENGTHENING: Using a wall or some other immoveable object, perform light strengthening exercises.

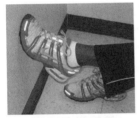
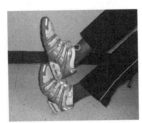

PLANATAR FLEXION
(foot down)

DORSIFLEXION
(resist upward motion with the other foot)

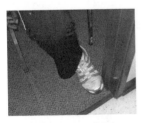
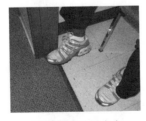

EVERSION (out)

INVERSION (in)

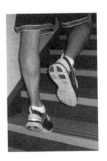

3. STEPS: Stand in front of a set of stairs, and slowly step up onto the first step with the leg you plan to exercise, and then step up with the other

leg. Once both feet are on the step, slowly step back down with the nonexercising foot first, keeping your weight on the exercising foot. Relax and take a deep breath. This is one repetition. Do three sets of ten repetitions, on each leg, a day.

4. SINGLE-LEG BALANCE: Stand and try to balance on the exercising leg without any support (keep a chair next to the nonexercising leg to use for balance as needed). Hold this position for 30 seconds, then relax and take a deep breath. This is one repetition. Do two sets of three repetitions for each leg, each day. Once the exercise becomes easier to do with the exercising foot flat on the floor, try lifting the heel slightly off the floor. Also, do this exercise with your eyes open at first. As it gets easier, try the exercise with your eyes closed. Once that gets easier, do this exercise while standing on a folded towel or pillow.

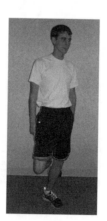 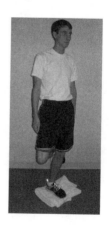

5. DYNAMIC SINGLE-LEG BALANCE: This is very similar to the single-leg balance exercise in step 4, except while balancing on one leg, reach in front of you with the arm on the same side as

the exercising leg and allow the exercising knee to bend. Balance, reach out, hold for 5 seconds, then slowly return to the starting position, relax, and take a deep breath. This is one repetition. Do two sets of ten repetitions for each leg, each day. Once this becomes easier, try reaching across your body for the chair next to your nonexercising leg.

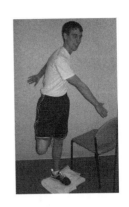

6. HOPPING/JUMPING: Once you can do exercises 1–5 without much of a problem, try hopping (initially on both legs, then later only on one leg) across the room and back. Then repeat the exercise using the other leg. This is one repetition. Do two sets of three repetitions for each leg, each day. Make sure that the path you are taking is free of obstacles or loose carpeting or rugs. Once the exercise becomes easier, perform the exercise jumping as high as you can each time you move forward, as opposed to just hopping. Make sure that you land softly, bending at both the ankle and the knee. Avoid landing hard on your feet and heels.

Phases 4 and 5 ankle rehabilitation consists of gradual return to jogging, running, jumping rope, agility training drills, noncontact activities and drills, and finally return to participation. Once you are completely free of pain, swelling, or other symptoms, and you can perform the phase 1 through 3 exercises well, you are ready to move into phase 4 and gradually return to training and participation. Particular attention should be given to the balance exercises in steps 4 and 5. But the most important thing to remember is that you continue to be at risk for reinjuring your ankle. So, progress gradually and at your own pace.

Figure 20: Exercises for Plantar Fasciitis

Stretching

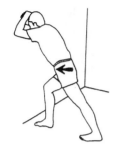

1. STANDING GASTROCNEMIUS (CALF) STRETCH: Standing in front of a wall, place both hands on the wall and step back with the leg you are planning to stretch, keeping the other, supporting leg forward and bent at the knee. Turn the foot of your stretching leg inward (so that your toes are pointing at the wall). Keep the stretching leg's heel on the floor. Now, slowly lean forward and feel the gentle stretch in the back of your calf. Hold the stretch for 15–30 seconds. Then relax and take a deep breath. This is one repetition. Do several sets of three repetitions for each leg, each day.

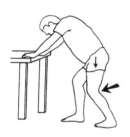

2. STANDING SOLEUS STRETCH: This exercise is performed the same way as the standing calf stretch in step 1, except you keep the stretching leg's knee slightly bent. You will feel the stretch in a different area in the back of your calf. Once again, it is important to keep the stretching leg's heel to the floor and your foot turned slightly inward.

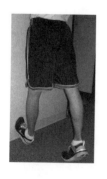

3. PLANTAR FASCIA STRETCH: Place the affected foot at a 45 degree angle at the bottom of a wall with the toes pushed upward; slowly move the hips toward the wall, feeling the stretch in the calf and sole of the foot. Hold for 15 seconds. Repeat five times and perform this two times a day.

4. ICE MASSAGE: Roll the foot over a can of frozen orange juice with pressure just in front of the heel. Massage for 5–10 minutes one or two times per day.

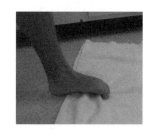

Strengthening

TOE CURLS: Place a towel on a hardwood or linoleum floor with the affected bare foot about two thirds on the towel. Forcibly curl the toes, wrinkling the towel. Perform three sets of ten repetitions. When this becomes easy, place a book on the towel to add more resistance.

Glossary

A

Abduction: Joint motion moving away from the midline.

Achilles tendon: The large tendon in the back of the heel.

Anemia: Low blood count; often from iron deficiency or blood loss.

Anterior: Toward the front.

Apophysis: Secondary growth center at the attachment site of major tendons around major joints.

Apophysitis: Inflammation of the apophysis in growing athletes.

AVN: Avascular necrosis; bone that loses its blood supply and dies.

Avulsion: Identifies when something is pulled off. A type of "chip" fracture.

B

Boxer's fracture: Fracture of the metacarpal (knuckle) of the small finger of the hand.

Burner: Injury to the brachial plexus in the shoulder causing burning sensation in the shoulder and arm.

Bursa: Potential space that allows tendons, muscles, and skin to slide past each other in a frictionless manner. Can be found throughout the body.

Bursitis: Inflammation of a bursa; from trauma or repetitive-friction causes.

C

Carpal bones: The eight bones in the wrist.

Cervical spine: The neck, consisting of eight vertebrae.

Crepitus: Grinding that can be felt or heard in a tendon or joint.

D

DIP: Distal interphalangeal joint; the finger joint closest to the finger tip.

Diskitis: Infection of the intervertebral disc.

Dislocation: Out of place; pertaining to a joint.

E

EIA: Exercise-induced asthma.

EIB: Exercise-induced bronchospasm or wheezing.

Extension: Movement of a joint moving away from the body or straightening.

Extrinsic: Outside the body.

Extrusion: Tooth movement in the direction of eruption.

F

First CMC: The carpal-metacarpal joint of the thumb.

Flexion: Joint motion in which the joint moves closer to the body.

Fracture: Broken bone or tooth.

H

Handlebar palsy: Injury to the ulnar nerve in the palm caused by a bicycle's handlebar.

Hyperpronation: Dynamic flattening of the feet in walkers or runners. Also known as overpronation.

I

Inferior: Below or under.

Intrinsic: Within the body.

Intrusion: Movement of a tooth back into the bone.

Ischemia: Lack of blood flow.

Ischium: The pelvic bone in the buttocks or bottom that is the upper attachment site for the hamstring muscle.

K

Kinetic chain: A term coined by Ben Kibler identifying the series of joint motions to generate a sport or occupational joint motion.

L

Lateral: Outside or farther from the midline.

Lisfranc joint: The collection of the joints in the middle portion of the foot between the tarsal and metatarsal joints approximately in the middle portion of the arch.

Lumbar spine: The lower back, consisting of five vertebrae.

Luxation: A term for partial dislocation; aka, subluxation; a term applied to partially dislocated teeth.

M

Malocclusion: Abnormal alignment of teeth.

Medial: Inside or closer to the midline.

Meniscus: The two crescent cartilage cushions in the knee.

Metacarpal: A bone that connects the wrist to the knuckle of a finger.

Migraine Headache: Identifies a classification of a headache characterized by acute onset of a throbbing one-sided headache associated with nausea, light sensitivity and occasionally tearing and nasal congestion.

N

NSAID: Nonsteroidal anti-inflammatory drugs; e.g., naproxen, ibuprofen, etc.

P

PIP: Proximal interphalangeal joint; the finger joint closer to the knuckle.

Posterior: Behind or toward the back.

PRICEMM: A mnemonic for early management of injuries that stand for protection, relative rest, ice, compression, elevation, medications, and modalities.

Pronation: The motion of the forearm in which the palm rotates down or the foot becomes more flat.

R

Reduction: Placing a dislocated joint or broken bone back in place.

Rotator cuff: The four stabilizing muscles of the shoulder; these muscles form a continuous tendon over the upper portion of the humerus or arm bone; these muscles are the supraspinatus, infraspinatus, teres minor and subscapularis.

S

Salter Harris fracture: A classification system for growth plate fractures in children grading them from 1 through 5 in ascending order of severity.

Scapula: The shoulder blade.

Scapular stabilizers: The muscles around the shoulder blade that support the shoulder blade when the arm and shoulder is moved through its wide range of motion.

Sciatica: A term for irritation of the sciatic nerve in the buttocks and leg. Manifested by chronic aching pain the radiates from the buttocks down the leg and is aggravated by sitting or coughing and sneezing. Sciatic pain is the same pain that one with a herniated disc will experience.

Spondylolisthesis: A slippage of one vertebral body on another, usually in the lower back and associated with spondylolysis.

Spondylolysis: A fracture of the pars interarticularis of the vertebral body; usually a stress fracture; spondylolysis on both sides at the same level may result in slippage (spondylolisthesis).

Sprain: Injury of a muscle; graded 1–3.

Stinger: *See* burner.

Strain: Injury to a ligament; graded 1–3.

Subluxation: Partial dislocation; this may be transient or a joint or tendon may be stuck in this partially dislocated position.

Suprascapular nerve: A nerve on the top of the shoulder that is often injured by stretching from a backpack or a direct blow on top of the shoulder as with a lacrosse stick.

T

Turf toe: Injury to the big toe when it is hyperextended, often on artificial turf, injuring the ball joint of the big toe.

U

URI: Upper respiratory infection; a cold.

V

Valgus: Movement or posturing of a limb in which the part farther from the center of the body is farther from the midline.

Valsalva: The act of increasing the pressure in the abdomen or chest as when coughing, straining to have a bowel movement, or lifting an object without breathing.

Vascular: Pertaining to blood flow.

Bibliography

Hutchinson, M. R., "Cheerleading Injuries: Patterns, Prevention, Case Reports." *Phys Sportsmed*; 25, no. 9 (1997): 83–90.

LaBotz, M. "Coping with Patellofemoral Syndrome." *Phys Sportsmed* 32, no. 7 (2004): 22-31.

Mellion, M. B., W. M. Walsh, C. Madden, M. Putukian, and G. L. Shelton. *Team Physician's Handbook.* 3rd ed. Philadelphia: Hanley & Belfus, Inc., 2002.

O'Connor, F. G., P. St. Pierre, W. Wilder. *Just the Facts in Sports Medicine.* New York: McGraw-Hill, 2005.

Noakes, T. *Lore of running,* 3rd ed., Leisure Press, Champaign, IL, 1991.

Index

Abdomen
  misdiagnoses in, 25
  trauma to, 76–77
Abdominal injuries, hockey and, 156
Abduction, 32
  shoulder, 172, 172
*About.com—Sports Medicine and
  Health*, 168
Acetaminophen, 10, 19
  for acromioclavicular sprain, 55
  for back pain, 80
  for cauliflower ear, 42
  for exertion-induced migraine, 37
  for knee arthritis pain, 109
  for sciatica, 83
  for subungual hematomas, 72
  for tennis elbow, 60
Acetic acid, swimmer's ear treatment
  with, 148, 149
Achilles tendinosis, 119–120
Achilles tendon, 119
  baseball playing and rupture of, 129
  basketball and problems with, 134
  martial arts/wrestling and problems
    with, 162
  running sports and problems with,
    133
Achilles tendon injuries
  bicycling and, 139
  tennis and, 151
  types of, 119–120
Achilles tendonitis exercises, 202–203
AC joint, 54

Acromioclavicular (AC) injuries
  basketball and, 134
  skiing, snowboarding and, 135
  volleyball and, 157
Acromioclavicular (AC) sprains
  soccer and, 143
  treatment of, 54–55
Acromioclavicular (AC) strains, soccer
  and, 143
Acromioclavicular (AC) tears, football,
  rugby, lacrosse and, 145
Acromion, 52
Active hamstring stretch, 180, 180,
  182, 182, 188, 188, 191, 191
Acute clots, in lungs, 13
Acute illness, resuming exercise after,
  15–16
Acute injuries
  prevention of, 14–15
  PRICEMM and, 16–18
  volleyball and, 156
Adhesive capsulitis, 57–58
Aerobic training, diabetics and, 4
Aikido injuries, 162–164
Airway resistance, 11
Albuterol, 12
Allergies, 12
Altitude sickness
  skiing, snowboarding and, 135
  symptoms of, 136
Aluminum acetate otic, swimmer's ear
  treatment with, 148–149
Amenorrhea, female athletes and, 3

American Academy of Family Practice (AAFP), 146
American Academy of Pediatrics (AAP), 146
American Association of Cheerleading Coaches and Advisors, 166
American College of Sports Medicine (ACSM), 146
American Medical Society for Sports Medicine (AMSSM), 146
  Web site of, 168
American Orthopedic Society of Sports Medicine (AOSSM), 146
Amitriptyline, 38
Anemia
  exercise and pregnant women with, 7
  shortness of breath during exercise and, 11–12
Anesthetics, for knee arthritis pain, 109
Aneurysms, 38
Angina, abdominal pain and, 79
Ankle braces, 117, 118
Ankle injuries
  baseball playing and, 129
  football, rugby, lacrosse and, 146
  hockey and, 154
Ankle pain, physician consultation about, 118–119
Ankle range of motion, 198–199
Ankle rehabilitation, 198–201
  phase 1 of, 198, 198
  phases 2 and 3 of, 198
  phases 4 and 5 of, 201
Ankle sprains, 116–117
  basketball and, 134
  cheerleading and, 166
  martial arts, wrestling and, 162
  rehabilitation phases for, 198

skiing, snowboarding and, 135
soccer and, 143
tennis and, 151
volleyball and, 156
Ankylosing spondylitis, 81–82
Anterior cruciate ligament (ACL), 101–104
  female athletes and injury to, 2
  sprains, 101–104
    preventing, 104
Anterior hip pain, 91
  causes of, 93
Anterior knee pain, causes of, 97
Antihistamines, 10
Apophysis, 29
Apophysitis, 29–31
Aquatic athletes, swimmer's ear and, 148–149
Arches, sore and tired, 122–125
Arch heights, shoe types and, 124
Arthritis, 65
  anterior cruciate ligament sprains and, 103–104
  anterior knee pain and, 97
  back pain and, 81–82
  corticosteroid injections and, 20
  knee, 107–110
  nonsteroidal anti-inflammatories and, 19
  in thumb, 69
Arthroscopy, 103, 106, 107, 110
Asthma, 12, 13
  exercise-induced, 11
Athletic Advisor, The, 167
Athletic pubalgia, 89
Athletic shoes, 124
Automated external defibrillator (AED)
  baseball games and readiness of, 129

hockey and readiness of, 156
Avascular necrosis (AVN), 92–93
Avulsion, 43, 44
Avulsion fracture, hip pain and, 91
Axe kicks, 163

Backhand form (tennis), elbow injuries
and, 151
Back injuries
boxing and, 161
cheerleading and, 166
football, rugby, lacrosse and, 145
hockey and, 155
martial arts, wrestling and, 162
rowing and, 159
skiing, snowboarding and, 135
tennis and, 151, 152
Back pain, 79–81
acute, exercises for, 179
bicycling and, 139
in children, 27–29
core stability and, 84–85
evaluation of, 81
golf and, 149
martial arts, wrestling and, 162
volleyball and, 158
x-rays for, 81–82
Backstroke, swimming injuries and,
147
Bacterial infections, wrestling and, 165
Balance, core stability and, 84
Ball machines (tennis), 152
"Bamboo spine," 82
Baseball, common injuries in, and
prevention of, 128–130
Baseball games, safety tips for,
129–130
Basketball injuries
common, 134
prevention of, 134–135

Batters, protection for, 129
Belly breathing, stitches and, 78
Bench press activities, young athletes
and, 32
Benzoin, tincture of, hot spots treated
with, 23
Beta blockers, 38
"Bible method," ganglion cysts and, 67
Bicycle measuring systems, 142
Bicycles
design types, 141
size and dimension issues related to,
142–143
Bicycling equipment, injury prevention
and choices related to, 140–143
Bicycling injuries
common, 139
prevention of, 139–140
Bindings, ski, 136
Blisters, treating, 22–23
Blood clots, calf pain and, 115–116
Bone scans, 29
Bony spine, 83
Boot designs, skiing, 136
Boutonnière deformity, 71
Boxer's fracture, 161
martial arts, wrestling and, 163
Boxing injuries, common, 160–162
Boys, soccer injuries among, 143
Brace lifts, calf pain treatment and,
115
Braces, 109
ankle, 117, 118
counterforce, 152
knee, 102, 103, 106
Brachial plexus, burners and, 48, 49
Breakaway bases, 130
Breaststroke, swimming injuries and,
147

Breaststroker's knee, in swimmers, 101, 147

Breath and breathing
shortness of, during exercise, 11–12
stitches and, 78

Bridge, 181, *181*

Bridging, 85

Buckle fractures, 26

Buddy taping, for jammed fingers, 70–71

Budesonide, 12

Burners, 48–49
football, rugby, lacrosse and, 145
martial arts, wrestling and, 162

Burroughs, Susan, 85

Bursas, 52, 63

Bursitis, 89
anterior knee pain and, 97
corticosteroid injections and, 20
of the elbow, 63

Butterfly, swimming injuries and, 147

Calcium channel blockers, 38

Calcium supplements, 114

Calf pain, 114–116
causes of, 115–116

Calf strains
basketball and, 134
running sports and, 133
tennis and, 151

Calluses, managing, 23

Caloric intake, for female athletes, 3

Camphor, 18

Cancer, back pain and, 81

Cane range of motion, *176*
for shoulder, 176

Canes, 109

Capsaicin, 18

Cardiac-related chest pain, 13

Carpal bones, 65

Carpal tunnel syndrome
corticosteroid injections and, 20
explanation of, 67–68
treatment of, 68–69

Cartilage, knee arthritis and, 107

Cartilage tears
description of, 105–106
treatment of, 106–107

Catback, *179*
for acute back pain, 179

Catchers, protection for, 129

Cauliflower ear
rugby and, 145
treatment of, 42–43

Cellulites, wrestling and, 165

Central (or white-white) meniscal tears, 106

Central slip injuries, 71

Cervical spine injuries, hockey and, 155

Chair lifts, 190, *190*

Cheerleading
injuries related to, 165–167
safety recommendations for, 166–167

Chest guards, boxing and, 161

Chest injuries
boxing and, 161
hockey and, 156
martial arts, wrestling and, 162
skiing, snowboarding and, 135

Chest pain, exercise and, 12–14

Chest wall, blunt injuries to, 76

Children
anterior knee pain in, 97
apophysitis in, 29–31
back pain in, 27–29
commotio cordis in, 129
fractures unique to, 26–27
heading the soccer ball by, 144

patellofemoral pain syndrome in, 100
weight lifting and, 31–32
Chin tucks, 170
Chondroitin, osteoarthritis pain and, 110
Chondromalacia patellae, 98
Cho-Pat brace, 30
Chronic medical conditions, sports, exercise and, 3–4
Chronic traumatic synovitis, martial arts, wrestling and, 163
City (cruiser) bikes, 141
Clavicle fracture, hockey and, 156
Cleaning, skin injuries, 21
Clothing. *See also* Shoes
  bicycling, 141
  cold-weather exercise and, 137
  hot weather exercise and, 138
Coaches, cheerleading, 166, 167
Colds, exercise and, 7–10
Cold weather, safe exercising during, 137
Collisions
  bicycling and, 139
  soccer and, 143
Collodian, 42
Commotio cordis
  baseball playing and, 129
  hockey and, 156
Compartment syndrome, 112, 114
Complex regional pain syndrome (CRPS), 26
Compression, 17
Compression wrap, for hamstring, 188
Concussions, 37, 41
  basketball and, 134
  bicycling and, 139
  boxing and, 160, 161
  cheerleading and, 166

football, rugby, lacrosse and, 145
hockey and, 155
martial arts, wrestling and, 162, 163
signs and symptoms of, 34–35
skiing, snowboarding and, 135
treatment of, 35–36
Conditioning programs
  baseball games and, 129–130
  skiing, snowboarding and, 136
Contagiosum, wrestling and, 165
Contusions
  martial arts, wrestling and, 162
  soccer and, 143
Cooling, injuries and, 17
Core flexibility exercises, 180
Core stability, 83–85
Core strengthening exercises, 181
  for back, 80, 81
    tennis and, 153
  rowing and, 159
Corticosteroid injections
  explanation of and risks associated with, 20–21
  for plantar fasciitis, 121
Corticosteroids, 20
  for knee arthritis pain, 109
Cortisone, 20
  injections of, for tennis elbow, 61
Coughing, 13
Counterforce braces, tennis and, 152
Cowboy collars, 49
Cramps
  exercise-induced, 10–11
  treatment and prevention of, 10–11
Crepitus, 105
Cromolyn, 12
Crunch, 181, *181*
Crutches, 120
Cubital tunnel syndrome, treatment of, 63–65

Curveballs, Little League elbow and, 130, 131
Cuts
  basketball and, 134
  bicycling and, 139
  boxing and, 161
  facial, 39
  martial arts, wrestling and, 162
  treating, 21–22
Cycling, diabetics and, 4

Deconditioning, shortness of breath during exercise and, 11–12
Degenerative joint disease (DJD), 107, 110
Deltoid ligament sprain, hockey and, 154
Dental injuries, 41, 43–44
  baseball and, 129
  basketball and, 134
  boxing and, 161
  hockey and, 155
  martial arts, wrestling and, 162, 163
DeQuervain's tenosynovitis, 65, 66
Dexamethasone, 20
Diabetes, sports, exercise and, 3–4
Diaphragm, 78
Differential diagnosis, 25
Disk herniation, 82–83, 159
Diskitis, in children, 27, 28
Dislocation, 32
Distal interphalangeal joint (DIP), 70, 71
Diving injuries, common, 147–148
Donut pads, heel pad contusions and, 121
Dorsal foot injuries, hockey and, 154
Dorsiflexion, 199
  for ankle rehabilitation, 199
  strengthening, 195, 195

Double leg knee-chest stretching, 179
Dressings, for skin injuries, 21–22
Dugout, protection for players in, 130
Dynamic single-leg balance, 200, 200–201

Ear covers, for baseball batters, 129
Ear injuries, martial arts, wrestling and, 162
Early pronation, 125
Ear plugs, 149
Ear protection, martial arts, wrestling and, 163
Eating disorders, cheerleaders and, 167
Eccentric training, 31
Effusion, 108
Elbow, bursitis of, 63
Elbow dislocations, football, rugby, lacrosse and, 145
Elbow flexor stretch, 178, 178
Elbow injuries
  boxing and, 161
  cheerleading and, 166
  golf and, 149
  golfer's elbow, 152
  Little League elbow, 128, 130–131
  martial arts, wrestling and, 162
  tennis and, 151
Electrical nerve studies, volleyball-related suprascapular nerve injury diagnosis and, 157
Electrical stimulation, 18
Electrocardiograms, 13
Electromyogram (EMG), carpal tunnel syndrome and, 68–69
Eletriptan, 37
Elevation, 17
Emergency medical services (EMS), baseball games and readiness of, 129

Emphysema, 13

Environmental conditions, running clothing/accessories and, 134

Equipment
cheerleading, 167
football, rugby, lacrosse, 146
hockey, 153–154
preventing sports-related injuries and choices related to, 14–15

Ergonomics, preventing neck injuries and, 46

Esophageal reflux, 13

Eversion, *199*
for ankle rehabilitation, 199

Exercise-induced asthma (EIA), 11

Exercise-induced bronchospasm (EIB), 11, 12

Exercise(s), 169–203
Achilles tendonitis, 202–203
acute back pain, 179
ankle rehabilitation, 198–201
back pain and, 80
chest pain and, 12–14
cold or flu and, 7–10
core flexibility, 180
core strengthening, 181
diabetes, high blood pressure, and chronic medical conditions, 3–4
golfer's elbow, 178
groin strain, 182–183
hamstring, 188–190
neck, 169–171
patellofemoral, 191–193
for plantar fasciitis, 196–197
pregnancy and, 5–7
quad, 186–187
resumption of, after injury or illness, 15–16
scapular, 173
for shin splints, 194–195

shortness of breath during, 11–12
shoulder, 172, 174–176
snapping hip, 184–185
tennis and intensity, duration, and frequency of, 152
for tennis elbow, 60, 177

Exertional compartment syndrome (ECS), 26
calf pain and, 115

Exertional migraine headaches, 37–38

Extension, female athletes and, 2

Extensor carpi radialis brevis (ECRB), 59

Extensor stretch, *177*
for tennis elbow, 177

External obliques, 76

External rotation of shoulder, 172, *172*

Extrinsic issues, overuse injuries and, 14

Extrusion, 43

Eye damage, facial injuries and, 39–40

Eye injuries
baseball playing and, 129
basketball and, 134
boxing and, 160
football, rugby, lacrosse and, 145
hockey and, 155
martial arts, wrestling and, 162
treatment of, 40–41

Eyewear, bicycling, 141

Face masks
football, rugby, lacrosse, 146
hockey, 154

Facet joints, 28

Facet pain, 80

Facial injuries, 39–40
baseball playing and, 129
basketball and, 134
boxing and, 160

hockey and, 155
martial arts, wrestling and, 162
skiing, snowboarding and, 135
Fainting, 11
Fall onto the outstretched hand
(FOOSH), 65
Falls
bicycling and, 139
soccer and, 143
Fatigue, overtraining and, 23–24
Fatigued muscles, spasms, cramps and,
10–11
Fatigue theory, about stress fractures,
113
Fat pad atrophy (or insufficiency), 122
Female athletes, prevention of sports
injuries in, 2–3
Female athlete triad
cheerleaders and, 167
three diagnoses within, 3
Femoral neck stress fractures, 92
Fever, 7
Fighting, hockey culture and, 153
Finger injuries
baseball playing and, 129
basketball and, 134
jammed fingers, 70–72
martial arts, wrestling and, 163
skiing, snowboarding and, 135
volleyball and, 158
First aid, 16
First CMC, 69
Fitness, for knees, 109
Flare-ups, knee arthritis, 108
Flat plantar arch, 122
Flat planus arches, shoes and, 124
Flexibility
core flexibility exercises, 180
core stability and, 84
Flexion, 44

Floater serve (volleyball),
suprascapular nerve injury and,
158
Flu, exercise and, 7–10
Fluticasone, 12
Flying kicks, 163
Foam boots, martial arts, wrestling
and, 163
Football injuries
common, 144–146
prevention of, 146
Foot care, diabetics, exercise and, 4
Foot injuries
football, rugby, lacrosse and, 146
volleyball and, 157
FootSmart Web site, 168
Footwear, personalized approach to,
123
Forearm bands, volleyball and, 158
Forearm pads, martial arts, wrestling
and, 163
Forehand mechanics (tennis), wrist
injuries and, 152
Forward elevation, of shoulder, 172,
172
Fractures
boxer's fracture, 161, 163
in children, 26–27
facial, 39
jaw, 41
rib, 76
stress, 112–114, 157, 163
wrist, 65
Frame sizes, bicycle, 142
Freestyle stroke, swimming injuries
and, 147
Friction blisters, 22
Friction massage, 177, 178
for golfer's elbow, 178
for tennis elbow, 177

Frostbite, preventing, 137
Frozen shoulder, 57–58
  corticosteroid injections and, 20
Fungal infections, wrestling and, 165

Gallbladder, 77
Gamekeeper's thumb
  hockey and, 156
  volleyball and, 158
Ganglion cysts, 66–67
  corticosteroid injections and, 20
Gastrocnemius stretch, standing, 194,
  196, 202
Gastrointestinal illnesses, exercise and,
  8
Gel-based heel cups, fat pad atrophy
  and, 122
Gender, soccer injuries and, 143
Genital trauma
  bicycle seat design and prevention
    of, 141
  bicycling and, 139
Gilmore's groin, 89, 90
  running sports and, 133
Girls, soccer injuries among, 143
Gloves
  bicycling, 141
  boxing, 161
  hockey, 156
  martial arts, wrestling and, 163
Glucocorticoids, 20
Glucosamine, osteoarthritis pain and,
  110
Goalkeepers (hockey), safety issues for,
  154
Goals, movable, soccer injuries and,
  144
Golf cart safety, 150
Golfer's elbow, 129, 152
  corticosteroid injections and, 20

exercise for, 178
treatment for, 62
volleyball and, 158
Golfing injuries
  common, 149
  prevention of, 150
Gout, olecranon bursa and, 63
Greenstick fracture, 26
Groin, misdiagnoses in, 25
Groin cups, martial arts, wrestling and,
  163
Groin protectors, boxing and, 161
Groin pull, treatment of, 88–89
Groin strain
  exercises for, 182–183
  hockey and, 154
  running sports and, 133
Growth centers, 26–27, 29
Growth plate fractures, in children,
  26, 27
Gymnastic routines, in cheerleading,
  166

Hamate, 149
Hamstring exercises, 188–190
Hamstring pulls, 95–96
Hamstring sleeve, 188
Hamstring strains, running sports and,
  133
Hamstring strength, improving, in
  women athletes, 3
Hand fractures
  boxing and, 161
  martial arts, wrestling and, 163
Hand injuries
  basketball and, 134
  football, rugby, lacrosse and, 145
  golf and, 149
  hockey and, 156
  rowing and, 160

skiing, snowboarding and, 135
volleyball and, 158
Handlebar height, bicycle, 143
Handlebar palsy, bicycling and, 139
Headaches, 36–38
migraine, 37–38
Headgear, boxing, 161
Heading the soccer ball, controversy
around, 144
Head injuries, 34–44
basketball and, 134
bicycling and, 139
boxing and, 160, 161
cheerleading and, 166
football, rugby, lacrosse and, 145
hockey and, 155
martial arts, wrestling and, 162, 163
skiing, snowboarding and, 135
soccer and, 144
Headlights (or headlamps), bicycling,
141
Head protection, martial arts,
wrestling and, 163
Healing, PRICEMM and, 16–18
Heart, 77
Heartburn, 13, 14
Heart problems, shortness of breath
during exercise and, 11–12
Heart-related chest pain, 13
Heat
for groin pull, 88
for neck injuries, 45
Heat cramps, 138
Heat exhaustion, 138
Heat injury, fever and, 7
Heatstroke, 138
Heel cups, heel pad contusions and,
121
Heel fat pad atrophy, 121
Heel lifts

Achilles tendon injuries and, 120
calf pain treatment and, 115
Heel pad contusions, 120, 121
Heel pain, 120–122
Heel problems
basketball and, 134
bicycling and, 139
running sports and, 133
Heel raise, 202, 202
Heel slide, 189, 189
Helmets
bicycling, 140–141
hockey, 154
skiing and, 136
Hematomas
eye, 40
septal, 39
subungual, 72–73
Hernias, 89
Herniated disks, 81
in children, 27
hockey and, 155
Herpes, wrestling and, 165
High blood pressure, sports, exercise
and, 3–4
High plantar arch, 122
Hip abductor strengthening, 185, 185
Hip adductor stretch, 182, 182
Hip contusions, football, rugby,
lacrosse and, 145
Hip flexions strengthening, 185, 185
Hip flexor stretch, 180, 180, 184, 184
Hip guards, football, rugby, lacrosse,
146
Hip pain, 90–93
causes of, 90–91
Hips, popping, snapping, and crackling
in, 94–95
Hockey equipment certification
(HECC), 154

Hockey injuries, common, 153–156

Hook of the hamate injury, golf and, 149–150

Hopping, *201*
  Achilles tendonitis exercise and, 203
  for ankle rehabilitation, 201

Hot and humid weather, exercise safety and, 138–139

Hot spots, 22, 23

Humid weather. *See* Hot and humid weather

Hutchinson, M. R., 167

Hybrid bikes, 141

Hydration
  bicycling and, 140
  broken teeth and, 43
  cold or flu and, 7, 9
  cold weather exercise and, 137
  headache prevention and, 37
  hot and humid weather exercise and, 139
  pregnancy, exercise and, 6
  prevention of spasms or cramps and, 11

Hygiene, grappling sports and, 165

Hyperpronation, 125

Hypothermia, preventing, 137

Ibuprofen, 10, 17, 19
  for acromioclavicular sprain, 55
  for back pain, 80
  for cauliflower ear, 42
  for exertion-induced migraine, 37
  for ganglion cysts, 67
  for jammed fingers, 70
  for sciatica, 83
  for subungual hematomas, 72
  for tennis elbow, 60
  for wrist pain, 66

Ice, 17
  for groin pull, 88
  for impingement or tendonitis, 53
  for jammed fingers, 70
  for neck injuries, 45
  for sciatica, 83
  for snapping hip syndrome, 94
  for tennis elbow, 60
  for wrist pain, 66

Ice hockey, 153

Ice massage, *197*
  for plantar fasciitis, 121, 197

Iliac apophysitis, 30

Iliotialband Friction Syndrome of the knee, bicycling and, 139

Iliotibial band stretching, 30

Iliotibial tract (IT), 94

Illnesses, resuming sports and exercise after, 15–16

Impetigo, wrestling and, 165

Impingement, 53

Impotence
  bicycle seat design and prevention of, 141
  bicycling and, 139

Infections, rashes and, 164–165

Infectious mononucleosis, 8

Inferior vena cava, 77

Inflammation, 16

Infraspinatus muscle, 52

Inguinal canal, 89

Inguinal hernias, 89

Injuries
  resuming sports and exercise after, 15–16
  treatment of with over-the-counter (OTC) medications, 18–19

Inside elbow apophysitis, 130

Internal obliques, 76

Intestines, 77

Intrinsic issues, overuse injuries and, 14

Intrusion, 43

Inversion, *199*
    for ankle rehabilitation, 199

Inversion strengthening, 195, 195

Ischemia, 25

Ischium, 30

Isometric strengthening, for ankle rehabilitation, 199

Jammed fingers, 70–72

Jaw injuries, 41
    baseball and, 129
    basketball and, 134
    boxing and, 160, 161
    martial arts, wrestling and, 162, 163

Jersey finger, 71–72

Joint locks, 163

Jones, Caitlyn, 117

Judo injuries, 162–164

Jumping, *201*
    Achilles tendonitis exercise and, 203
    for ankle rehabilitation, 201

Jumping kicks, 163

Karate injuries, 162–164

Kevlar throat protectors, hockey and, 154

Keyboarding, carpal tunnel syndrome and, 67–68

Kibler, Ben, 128, 132

Kickboxing injuries, 162–164

Kidneys, 77
    nonsteroidal anti-inflammatories and, 19

Kidney stones, back pain and, 81

Kinetic chain, 128, 132

Knee braces, 106

Knee-chest stretching, *179*
    for acute back pain, 179

Knee guards, football, rugby, lacrosse and, 146

Knee injuries
    cheerleading and, 166
    football, rugby, lacrosse and, 145
    hockey and, 154
    physician consultations about, 104
    rowing and, 159
    skiing and, 136
    tennis and, 151
    volleyball and, 156

Knee pain, anterior, 97

Knees
    anterior cruciate ligament sprains in, 101–104
    arthritis in, 107–110
    baseball playing and sprains of, 129
    breaststroker's knee, 147
    crepitus in, 105
    medial collateral ligament sprains in, 100–101

Kung fu injuries, 162–164

Lacerations
    eye, 40
    facial, 39

Lacrosse injuries
    common, 144–146
    prevention of, 146

Lateral epicondylitis, 59

Layering clothing, cold weather exercise and, 137

Leg bones, stress fractures in, 112

Levator scapula, 132

Lightning safety tips, golf and, 150

Lisfranc joint injuries, football, rugby, lacrosse and, 146

Little League elbow, 31, 128, 130–131

Little League shoulder, 131–133
Liver, 77
    nonsteroidal anti-inflammatories
      and, 18–19
Longitudinal arch, 122
Loose shoulder, throwing athletes and,
    132
Lore of Running, The (Noakes), 78
Lower back injuries, golf and, 149
Lower extremity injuries, 87–125, 129
Lumbar spine stresses, minimizing, in
    young athletes, 31
Lungs, acute clots in, 13
Luxation, 43

Magnetic resonance imaging (MRI),
    29
    ankle pain and use of, 118
    avascular necrosis and, 93
    of intervertebral disks and soft
      tissues, 83
    meniscal tears and, 106
    stress fractures and, 92
    volleyball-related suprascapular
      nerve injury diagnosis and, 157
Mallet finger, 71
Malocclusion, 41
Martial arts injuries
    common, 162
    preventing, 163–164
Massage, 18
    for groin pull, 88
    for neck injuries, 45
    for tennis elbow, 61
Mau's syndrome, 97
Medial, 98
Medial collateral ligament (MCL),
    100–101
    breaststroke and, 147
    Little League elbow and, 130

Medial collateral ligament (MCL)
    injuries, hockey and, 154
Medial collateral ligament (MCL)
    sprains
    skiing, snowboarding and, 135
    soccer and, 143
    treatment of, 100–101
Medial collateral ligament (MCL)
    tears, football, rugby, lacrosse and,
    145
Medial elbow pain, volleyball and, 158
Medial epicondylitis, 62, 128
    tennis and, 152
Medial tibial stress syndrome (MTSS),
    111
Medications, 17
    for neck injuries, 45
Men, inguinal canal in, 89
Meniscal injuries
    football, rugby, lacrosse and, 145
    soccer and, 143
    tennis and, 151
Meniscal tears, 105
    types of, 106
Meniscus (menisci), functions of, 105
Menstrual irregularities, in female
    athletes, 3
Menthol, 18
Metacarpal phalangeal (MCP) joint,
    69, 73
Microfractures, 112
Migraine headaches, 37–38
Misdiagnosed sports injuries, 24–26
Mites, wrestling and infections from,
    165
Modalities, 18
Modified straight-leg raises (Muncie
    method), 193, *193*
Moisture, controlling, 23

Moisture-wicking garments, hot weather exercise and, 138

Moleskin doughnuts, for hot spots, 23

Molluscum, wrestling and, 165

Mononucleosis, 8

Morton's neuroma, corticosteroid injections and, 20

Mountain (all-terrain) bikes, 141

Mountain (all-terrain) biking, clothing for, 141

Mouthguards
boxing and, 161
football, rugby, lacrosse and, 146
hockey and, 154
martial arts, wrestling and, 163

Moviegoer's knee, 98

Muscle relaxants, for back pain, 80

Muscle spasms, treatment and prevention of, 10–11

Muscle strains
risk factors for, 95
treating, 95–96

Muscular core, components of, 83–84

Myocarditis, 8

Myositis ossificans, 97

Naproxen, 10, 17, 19
for acromioclavicular sprains, 55
for back pain, 80
for cauliflower ear, 42
for exertion-induced migraines, 37
for ganglion cysts, 67
for sciatica, 83
for subungual hematomas, 72
for tennis elbow, 60
for wrist pain, 66

Naratriptan, 37

National Electronic Injury Surveillance System, 145

National Federation of State High School Associations, 167

"Neck check" test
athletes with upper respiratory infection and, 8–9
resuming exercise after acute illness and, 15–16

Neck collars, 49

Neck exercises
strengthening, 171
stretching and range of motion, 169–170

Neck extension stretch, 170, *170*

Neck flexion stretch, 170, *170*

Neck injuries, 41, 44–49
bicycling and, 139
cheerleading and, 166
football, rugby, lacrosse and, 145
hockey and, 155
martial arts, wrestling and, 162

Neck isometric extension, 171, *171*

Neck isometric flexion, 171, *171*

Neck isometric side-bending, 171, *171*

Neck pain, evaluation of, 47–48

Neck rotation stretch, 169

Neck side-bending stretch, 169, *169*

Neck sprains/strains, treatment of, 44–47

Nerve compression syndromes, rowing and, 160

Nerve entrapments, 25

Neurontin, 38

Neutral arches, 124

Noakes, Tim, 78

Nonsteroidal anti-inflammatory drugs (NSAIDs), 10, 17, 19
for back pain, 80
for knee arthritis pain, 109

Normal plantar arch, 122

Nortriptyline, 38

Nosebleeds
  skiing, snowboarding and, 135
  treating, 38–39
Nose injuries
  basketball and, 134
  boxing and, 160, 161
  martial arts, wrestling and, 162

Olecranon bursa, 63
Orgasmic migraine headaches, 37
Orthopedic evaluation, for shoulder
    problems, 59
Orthotic inserts, 109, 112
  Achilles tendon and use of, 119
  arch health and, 123, 124, 125
Osgood-Schlatter disease, 29–30, 97,
    100
  soccer and, 143
Osteoarthritis (OA), 107
  anterior cruciate ligament sprains
    and, 103–104
  pain in, 108
Osteonecrosis, 92
Osteoporosis
  back pain and, 81
  female athletes and, 3
Outrigger (rowing), 159
Overhead strokes, shoulder and back
    injuries and, 152
Overload theory, about stress fractures,
    113
Over-the-counter (OTC) medications,
    injury treatment and, 18–19
Overtraining, 23–24
  bicycling and, 139
  boxing and, 161
  martial arts, wrestling and, 163
  running sports and, 133
  swimming injuries and, 146
Overuse injuries
  basketball and, 135

bicycling and, 139, 140
golf and, 149
in the neck, 46
prevention of, 14–15
rowing and, 159, 160
soccer and, 143
volleyball and, 156, 158

Padded fences, 130
Pain medications, for impingement or
    tendonitis, 53
Pain relief, 19
Pancreas, 77
Pars interarticularis, 28
  stress fracture of, 82
Patellar dislocations, football, rugby,
    lacrosse and, 145
Patellar tendonitis
  basketball and, 134
  bicycling and, 139
  martial arts, wrestling and, 162
  running sports and, 133
  volleyball and, 156–157
Patellar tracking, abnormal, risk factors
    for, 98
Patellofemoral exercises, 191–192
Patellofemoral pain syndrome (PFPS),
    97, 98–99
  basketball and, 134
  bicycling and, 139
  exercises for, 191
  in female athletes, 2
  martial arts, wrestling and, 162
  running sports and, 133
  soccer and, 143
  swimming and, 147
  treatment for, 99
Pelvic joint pain, 80
Pelvic stress fractures, 92
Pelvic tilt, 85, 181, *181*
Pendleton, Joyce, 53–54

Pendulum exercises, 55, 174, *174*
PEP program, 104
Peripheral (or red-red) meniscal tears, 106
Physes, 27
Physical therapy
    for Achilles tendon injuries, 119–120
    recovery with, 117–118
Phys Sportsmed, 167
Pilates, 85
Piriformis muscle stretching, 85
Piriformis (seated), 180, *180*
Pitch counts by age, recommendations related to, 131
Pitchers
    Little League elbow and, 130–131
    shoulder and elbow problems in, 128
Pitching, child safety and, 129
Plantar arches
    basketball and, 134
    bicycling and, 139
    running sports and, 133
    types of, 122
Plantar fascia, 121
    stretch for, 196, *196*
Plantar fasciitis, 120–121
    corticosteroid injections and, 20
    exercises for, 196–197
    volleyball and, 157
Plantar flexion, *199*
    for ankle rehabilitation, 199
Polypropylene socks, 23
Popeye arm, 63
Posterior capsule stretch, *176*
    for shoulder, 176
Posterior headaches, 38
Prednisone, 20
Pregnancy, exercise and, 5–7

Preparticipation physical examination (PPE), 146
Preseason conditioning, skiing, snowboarding and, 136
Press-up extension, *179*
    for acute back pain, 179
Prevention, of sports-related injuries, 14–15
PRICEMM, 16–18
    Achilles tendon injuries treatment and, 120
    ankle pain and, 118
    anterior cruciate ligament sprain treatment and, 102
    boxing-related injuries and, 161
    hamstring exercises and, 188
    heel pad contusions and, 121
    hip pain and, 90, 91
    knee arthritis treatment and, 108
    medial collateral ligament treatment and, 101
    medial tibial stress syndrome treatment and, 112
    meniscal tear treatment and, 106
    muscle strains and, 96
    patellofemoral pain syndrome and, 99
    phase 1 ankle rehabilitation and, 198
    quad exercises and, 186
    sprained ankle treatment and, 117
    stress fracture treatment and, 114
Pronation, 14, 124–125
Pronator strengthening, *178*
    for elbow, 178
Prone hip extensions, 189, *189*
Prone knee bends, 189, *189*
Prone or seated retraction, *173*
    of shoulder, 173
Prophylactic medications, 38

Propranolol, 38

Protection, 16–17

Protective equipment, martial arts and wrestling, 163

Proximal fibular fracture, hockey and, 154

Proximal interphalangeal (PIP) joint, 70, 71

Proximal tibial fractures, skiing, snowboarding and, 135

Puck, hockey, 153, 154

Pudendal neuropathy, bicycling and, 139

Puncture wounds, treating, 21–22

Pyramid building, in cheerleading, 166, 167

Quad exercises, 186–187

Quadriceps, 11
    contusions, 96–97
    isometric strengthening, 186, *186*
    pulls, 95–96
    stretch, 186, *186*
    wall slide, 187, *187*, 192, *192*

Quadriceps tendonitis
    basketball and, 134
    bicycling and, 139
    martial arts, wrestling and, 162
    running sports and, 133
    volleyball and, 157

Quadruped, 85, 181, *181*

Rackets, tennis, 152

Radiation injuries, to eyes, 40, 41

Rashes, wrestling and, 164–165

Rectus abdominus, 76

Reduction, 56

Red-white meniscal tears, 106

Reflective tape, bicycling and, 141

Reflex sympathetic dystrophy (RSD), 26

Rehabilitation. *See also* Exercise(s)
    arch health and, 125
    exercises, 18

Repetitive motions, carpal tunnel syndrome and, 67

Resistance training
    for children, 31
    diabetics and, 4

Respiratory problems, shortness of breath during exercise and, 11–12

Respiratory-related chest pains, 13

Rest, 17
    for athletes with upper respiratory infections, 9
    for groin pull, 88
    for neck injuries, 45

Retropatellar pain, 98

Ribs, injuries to, 76

Rib stress fracture, rowing and, 160

Road bikes, 141

Road rash
    basketball and, 134
    bicycling and, 139
    boxing and, 161
    martial arts, wrestling and, 162

Rotator cuff, 52
    cheerleading and strengthening of, 167
    strengthening exercises for, 55, 56, 132
    tennis and strengthening of, 153

Rotator cuff injuries
    baseball and, 132
    swimming and, 147
    tennis and, 152
    volleyball and, 157

Rotator cuff tendonitis, 52–54
    baseball and, 128
    golf and, 149

Rowing, competitive, 158–159

Rowing injuries, common, 158–160

Rugby College (England), 144
Rugby injuries
    common, 144–146
    prevention of, 146
Runners
    high-risk stress fractures in,
        112–113
    pronation in, 125
Runner's knee, 98
Running injuries
    common, 133
    prevention of, 133–134
Running shoes, choosing/replacing,
    134

Sacroiliac pain, 80
Saddle position, bicycle, 142
Saddle sores
    bicycling and, 139
    prevention of, 141
Safety
    cold weather exercise and, 137
    hot and humid weather exercising
        and, 138–139
Salicylates, 18
Salmeteral/Fluticasone, 12
Salter Harris fractures, 26
Scabies, wrestling and infections from,
    165
Scapholunate dislocation, 65
Scapula, 52
Scapular exercises, 173
Scapular stabilizers, 132
Sciatica, explanation of, 82
Sciatic nerve, 82–83
Scrapes
    basketball and, 134
    bicycling and, 139
    boxing and, 161
    martial arts, wrestling and, 162
    treating, 21–22

Self-reduction, of shoulder, 175, *175*
Separated shoulder, 55
Septal hematoma, 39
Serving (tennis), shoulder and back
        injuries and, 152
Sever's disease, 30
    soccer and, 143
Shibla, Dani, 100
Shields, martial arts, wrestling and,
    163
Shin guards, soccer and, 144
Shin pain, 111
Shin splints, 111–112, 113, 114
    basketball and, 134
    exercises for, 194–195
    running sports and, 133
    soccer and, 143
    tennis and, 151
Shock-absorbing mats, martial arts,
        wrestling and, 163
Shoes
    arch problems and, 122–125
    blister prevention and fitting of,
        22–23
    football, rugby, lacrosse, 146
    medial tibial stress syndrome and
        importance of, 111–112
    running, 134
    shock-absorbing, 109
    stability, 125
    volleyball and, 157
    well-fitting, tips for, 123
Shorts, bicycling, 141
Shoulder dislocation (or laxity), 55–57
Shoulder impingement, 52–54
Shoulder injuries
    boxing and, 161
    football, rugby, lacrosse and, 145
    golf and, 149
    hockey and, 155–156
    martial arts, wrestling and, 162

range of motion exercise after, 174
skiing, snowboarding and, 135
swimming and, 146, 147
tennis and, 151
volleyball and, 157
Shoulder instability, baseball and, 128
Shoulder pads, 49
football, rugby, lacrosse and, 146
Shoulder problems, surgeon consults
for, 58–59
Shoulder reduction, 175
Shoulders
Little League shoulder and,
131–133
strengthening exercises for, 132,
172
stretching exercises for, 176
Shoulder separations, 54, 58–59
Side-leaning iliotibial band stretch,
184, *184*, 191, *191*
Side leg lifts, 30
Side-lying leg raise, 183, *183*
Side stitches, 77–79
Sinding-Larsen-Johansson (SLJ)
syndrome, 29, 97, 100
Single-leg balance, 200, *200*, 203, *203*
Single leg knee-chest stretching, *179*
SITS muscles, 52
Sitting hamstring stretch, 182, *182*,
188, *188*, 191, *191*
Skates, hockey, 153
Skier's thumb, 69
Skiing injuries
common, 135
prevention of, 136
Skin blisters
basketball and, 134
bicycling and, 139
running sports and, 133
Skin injuries, treating, 21–22
Skin problems, wrestling and, 164–165

Sliders, Little League elbow and, 130,
131
Sliding injuries, baseball playing and,
128–129
Sliding techniques, proper, 130
Slipped rib, 76
Snapping hip
exercises for, 184
running sports and, 133
syndrome, 94–95
Snapping knee (ITB) syndrome,
running sports and, 133
Snowboarding injuries, prevention of,
136
Soccer injuries
common, 143–144
prevention of, 144
Socks, polypropylene, 23
Softball play, safety tips for, 129–130
Soleus stretch, standing, 194, 196, 202
Spinal cord, 79
Spinal stenosis, 81, 83
Spine, 79
Spinning kicks, 163
Spirit Rule Book, 167
Spleen, 77
Splints, 109
carpal tunnel syndrome and, 68
cubital tunnel syndrome and, 64
Spondylolisthesis, 27, 28, 80, 82, 83
hockey and, 155
rowing and, 159
Spondylolysis, 27, 28–29, 80, 82
hockey and, 155
rowing and, 159
swimming and, 147
Sports
pregnancy and, 5–7
returning to, after injury or illness,
15–16
Sports hernia, 89–90

Sports injuries
    in female athletes, 2–3
    misdiagnosed, 24–26
    treatment of with over-the-counter
      (OTC) medications, 18–19
Sportsman's hernia, 89, 90
Sports Medicine Advisor, online version
    of, 167
Sportsmetrics program, 104
Sports-related injuries, prevention of,
    14–15
Sprains
    ankles, 116–117
    football, rugby, lacrosse and, 145
    neck, 44–47
    wrist, 65
Stability shoes, 125
Stabilization of shoulder in prone, 173,
    173
Stab injuries, facial, 39
Standing gastrocnemius stretch, 194,
    194, 196, *196*, 202, *202*
Standing soleus stretch, 194, *194*, 196,
    196, 202, *202*
Steps, *187*, *193*, *199*
    for ankle rehabilitation, 199–200
    patellofemoral exercises on, 193
    quad exercises on, 187
Steroid flare, 20–21
Steroids, side effects with, 21
Sticks, hockey, 153
Stingers, 48–49
    martial arts, wrestling and, 162
Stitches, 77–79
Stomach, 77
Straight leg raise, 183, *183*, 187, *187*,
    192, *192*
Straining headache, 38
Strengthening
    for Achilles tendonitis, 202–203
    core strengthening exercises, 181

    for elbow, 178
    for groin pull, 88
    for hamstring, 189–190
    hip abductor and hip flexions, 185
    for patellofemoral pain syndrome,
      192–193
    for plantar fasciitis, 197
    quadriceps isometric strengthening,
      186
    for shin splint, 195
    for tennis elbow, 60
Stress fractures, 112–114
    basketball and, 134
    bicycling and, 139
    calf pain and, 115
    female athletes and, 3
    hip pain and, 92
    in leg bones, 112
    martial arts, wrestling and, 163
    running sports and, 133
    soccer and, 143
    symptoms of, 114
    treatment of, 114
    volleyball and, 157
Stress testing, 4, 13
Stretching, 18
    for Achilles tendonitis, 202
    bicycling and, 140
    cold weather exercise and, 137
    core flexibility exercises, 180
    for golfer's elbow, 178
    for groin pull, 88
    hamstring stretches, 188
    martial arts, wrestling and, 163
    for neck injuries, 45
    for patellofemoral pain syndrome,
      191–192
    for plantar fasciitis, 196–197
    quadriceps stretch, 186
    rowing and, 159
    for shin splint, 194

for shoulder, 176
snapping hip exercises, 184
for tennis elbow, 60
volleyball and, 157
Stretching Institute Web site, 168
Stroke mechanics, tennis, 153
Subluxation, 32
Subscapularis, 52
Subungual hematoma, 72–73
Sumatriptan, 37
Supinator strengthening, *177*
for tennis elbow, 177
Suprascapular nerve injuries, volleyball
and, 157
Supraspinatus muscle, 52
Surgery
for anterior cruciate ligament
sprains, 103
carpal tunnel syndrome and, 68–69
for degenerative joint disease, 110
for meniscal tears, 106
Swelling
compression and, 17
with wrist pain, 65
Swimmer's ear, 148–149
Swimming
common injuries with, 146–147
diabetics and, 4
injuries related to primary strokes
in, 147
Swing mechanics, golf and, 149
Swiss exercise ball, 85
Synovitis (chronic, traumatic), boxing
and, 161
Synovium, 107

Tae kwon do injuries, 162–164
"Talk test," pregnancy, exercise, and, 6
Temperature
cold weather exercise and, 137

fever and, 7
hot and humid weather exercise
and, 138–139
Tendinopathy, 52–53
Tendonitis, 53, 97
in Achilles tendon, 120
corticosteroid injections and, 20
swimming and, 147
wrist, 65–66
Tennis elbow
corticosteroid injections and, 20
exercises for, 177
explanation of, 59
treatment of, 60–61
Tennis elbow straps, 60–61
Tennis injuries
common, 150–152
prevention of, 152–153
Tennis rackets, 152
Teres minor, 52
Tetanus boosters, 22
Theater sign, 99
Therapeutic ultrasound, 18
Thigh contusions, hockey and, 154
Throat protectors, hockey and, 154
Throwing mechanics, proper, 132
Thumb injury, 69–70
Time-trial bikes, 141
Tizatriptan, 37
TMJ joint, injuries to, 41
Toe curls, *197*
for plantar fasciitis, 197
Tooth injuries, 43–44
Topical treatments, 18
Topiramate, 38
Torus fractures, 26
Touring bikes, 141
Towel stretch, *176*
for shoulder, 176
Transverse arch, 122

Transversus abdominus, 76, 77, 84

Trapezius stretch, 170, *170*

Traumatic injuries, baseball playing and, 128–129

Traumatic synovitis, boxing and, 161

Triamcinolone, 20

Triamcinolone acetonide, 12

Triangular fibrocartilage complex (TFCC), 65, 66

Triathlon bikes, 141

Tricyclic antidepressants, 38

Trigger fingers, 73–74
   golf and, 149

Triptans, 37

Trochanteric bursitis, 94
   running sports and, 133

Trunk injuries, 75–85
   boxing and, 161
   martial arts, wrestling and, 162
   skiing, snowboarding and, 135

Turf toe, football, rugby, lacrosse and, 146

Two-person reduction, 175, *175*

Two-person technique, for shoulder dislocation, 56

Tylenol, 10

Ulnar collateral ligament (UCL), 69

Ulnar collateral ligament (UCL) injuries, hockey and, 156

Ulnar collateral ligament (UCL) sprains
   boxing and, 161
   martial arts, wrestling and, 162

Ulnar collateral ligament (UCL) strains, 128

Ulnar neuropathy, bicycling and, 139

United States Tennis Association (USTA), 150

University of Michigan, Sports Medicine Health Topics, 167

Upper extremity injuries, 51–74

Upper humerus, 52

Upper respiratory infections (URI), exercise and, 7–10

USA Baseball Medical and Safety Advisory Committee, 131

USA Hockey, 154

Valgus, anterior cruciate ligament injuries and, 2

Valgus load, Little League elbow and, 130

Valproic acid, 38

Valsalva, 38

Vascular pinching, 25

Verapamil, 38

Viral infections, wrestling and, 165

Viscosupplements, for knee arthritis pain, 109–110

Vitamin C, stress fracture treatment and, 114

Vitamin D, stress fracture treatment and, 114

Vocal cord dysfunction (VCD), 12

Volleyball injuries, common, 156–158

Walkers, 109

Walking, diabetics and, 4

Wall climbs, 55, 174, *174*

Warts, wrestling and, 165

Water-repellant clothing, 137

Weather, running clothing/accessories and, 134

Web sites, sports information, 167–168

Weight lifting, children and, 31–32

Weight-lifting headache, 38

Wet bulb globe, 138

Wheezing, 13
Whiplash injury, treatment of, 44–47
Women
    inguinal canal in, 89
    volleyball, ACL injuries and, 157
Woods, Tiger, 149
Workplace injuries, in the neck, 46
Wounds, treating, 21–22
Wrestling, rashes and, 164–165
Wrestling injuries
    common, 162
    preventing, 163–164
Wrestling mats, disinfected, 165
Wrist, torus or buckle fractures in, 26
Wrist extensor strengthening, 177
Wrist flexor strengthening, 178, 178
Wrist injuries
    basketball and, 134
    bicycling and, 139
    boxing and, 161

football, rugby, lacrosse and, 145
golf and, 149
martial arts, wrestling and, 162
rowing and, 160
skiing, snowboarding and, 135
soccer and, 143–144
tennis and, 152
volleyball and, 158
Wrist pain, 65–66

X-rays
    ankle pain and, 118
    avascular necrosis and, 93
    back pain and, 81–82
    stress fractures and, 92

Youth baseball injuries,
        recommendations related to, 131

Zolmitriptan, 37